Ten children die each and every minute of every hour of every day, day in, day out, year in, year out, from communicable diseases that can be prevented by immunization. Five of these are from measles.

Ten children are handicapped each and every minute of every hour of every day, day in, day out, year in, year out, from communicable diseases that can be prevented by immunization. Five of these are from measles.

**Dr. Jacob John, Virologist
Christian Medical College
Vellore, South India
September 1979**

ISBN 1-894439-03-1
Printed and bound in Canada

© 2000 Kenneth C. Hobbs, O.Ont. MD
All rights reserved.

For all inquiries, or to order additional copies of this book, please contact:

Dr. Kenneth C. Hobbs
320 Lyndeview Drive, Whitby ON L1N 3A3
telephone: (905) 668-6258
fax: (905) 668-7142
e-mail: khobbs@sprint.ca

Design and production by:

Baird, O'Keefe
Publishing Inc.

Publication Specialists
(613) 831-7628
Gail Baird, Managing Editor
Wendelina O'Keefe, Creative Director

Canadian Cataloguing in Publication Data

Hobbs, Kenneth C.
  Diary of a miracle

ISBN 1-894439-03-1

  1.   Rotary International—History. 2. Measles vaccine—India—History. 3. Hobbs, Kenneth C. I. Title.

RA644.M5H62 2000   369.5'2   C00-900855-1

Dedication

This book is dedicated to the many Rotarians of South India. It is impossible to mention everyone who has contributed their efforts to make this miracle happen. I wish to express my gratitude not only to the Rotarians, along with their wives and children, but also to the Interactors and Rotoactors of South India.

However, in the early stages and throughout the life of this project, there was one Rotarian, along with his dear wife, who exemplified the true and devoted actions of "Service above Self." In this book, you will soon recognize the Chitales, and my admiration of them. If I had encountered any persons other than Krish and Susheila Chitale in September 1979, then perhaps this project would have ended at that stage. I thank them for being our friends.

For my wife, who played a very significant role. Her understanding of my commitment, and frustrations at various stages of indecisiveness, were most appreciated. She never hesitated to encourage me to continue on and complete my goal. Her presence on my travels around the world, showed that she believed in the basic principles of "Service above Self."

Hopefully, our four grandchildren will learn by our example, as we did from our parents. I pray that they will understand the fullest meaning of Rotary's motto of "Service above Self" as they grow, mature and become self-reliant in their quests of helping the less fortunate in our world's society.

Preface

In his book *Diary of a Miracle*, Dr Ken Hobbs describes the obstacles meted out by various Rotarians and Governmental agencies, for the successful, first implementation of the introduction of measles vaccine into India. He further describes the difficulties in phase one and phase two of this important historical first for the Rotarians of South India. Of the famous four questions under the "four way test" of Rotary, the last two questions of the text prove the vitality of the programme, vis-a-vis "Will it build GOODWILL and BETTER FRIENDSHIP?"; and "will it be BENEFICIAL to all CONCERNED?"

We are on the threshold of the 21st Century and India has already covered enough grounds towards immunization, thanks to Rotary by starting with the Red Measles Program. This stimulated the concept of Polio Plus in 1984. This program will hopefully eradicate polio from the world by the year 2005, the 100th anniversary of Rotary International.

Throughout the world, Ken's concern about children's health is something of a rare phenomenon.

In the Rotary world he is called the "father of the red measles immunization program." Only a few Rotarians could create this "Diary of a Miracle."

It was in the late 1970s, the Rotarians of RI Dist 707 Canada were brought together with Rotarians of Southern India by Rotary International. During 1978-79 Rotarian Dist. Governor Nominee Bernard Crookes of District 707, initiated conversations at the International Assembly in Boca Raton Florida with District Governor Nominee P.Jagadeersan of District

320 India. They decided on initiating some meaningful "Canada-India World Community Service Project." They decided to embark on introducing measles vaccine for the first time into India. Measles was indeed a dreaded killer in India, and was the third cause of blindness in children under the age of five.

Four Clubs in Toronto pledged financial support along with the Canadian International Development Agency and The Rotary Foundation. These funds provided for an initial 68,000-dose project to immunize children against red measles in the Madras area. This initial program expanded the following year into a 5.2 million-dose project, sponsored by a "Health Hunger and Humanity" grant from The Rotary Foundation, along with a grant from the Canadian Government through CIDA (Canadian International Development Agency).

The details of the arrival of the first shipment on September the 25, 1979 are described by Dr. Ken. However I must add that Rotarian N. Kumar did a tremendous amount of work in approaching the federal governmental officials in order to obtain the all-important Import Permit and Duty Exemption certificates. This was a tedious uphill task. Rotarian Kumar was successful and the 68,000 doses of measles vaccine were allowed into India. This was the first significant amount of red measles vaccine ever to be allowed into my country.

In 1983, Dr. Ken and myself were able to receive encouraging help and support from Dr. H.V. Hande, the Honorable Minister of Health and Welfare for the State of Tamil Nadu. This in itself was a first for all of India, if not in the whole Rotary world. For the first time, a combined committee was set up between Rotarians and State health officials to administer a State immunization program.

I met Dr. Ken Hobbs for the first time on Sept 14, 1979. His dedication and hard work in implementing this miracle inspired me very much. Since 1979 we have worked together on other social needs, details of which I list below:

- Child Trust Hospital is the only non profit pediatric hospital in the private sector in Madras (now called Chennai). Dr. Ken Hobbs was responsible for obtaining a US $608,000.00 grant from The Rotary Foundation. These funds supplied surgical, medical and other equipment for the hospital.

- The Rotary Worth Trust Project was a combined project with Dr. Ken spearheading the project. He was able to receive a US $93,000.00 grant from The Rotary Foundation, along with Can $75,000.00 from the Clubs of District 707. This training and rehabilitation project enabled handicapped persons to become self-sufficient

- Thanner Water Project—the city of Chennai has been suffering from severe water shortage. This project has revitalized some Temple water to once again act as aquifers and has recharged local wells with fresh potable water.

- Rehabilitation and Training for Disabled Persons—Dr. Ken's energy and knowledge has allowed the Rotary Club of Madras to receive a US $500,000.00 grant from The Rotary Foundation, to train, rehabilitate and employ handicapped persons. The first phase is concentrating on polio victims, who have never received any form of rehabilitation or training, in order to make them self-sufficient.

I would like to add my views and my personal feelings concerning Ken and Eva, and what this association means to me personally. With Dr. Ken, one point has been proven beyond any doubt. The world we live in may be large in area; however, when it comes to people, it is one big neighborhood. When I first went to receive Ken and Eva at the Madras airport on September 14, 1979, I was filled with apprehension about what kind of people I was going to work with. I am sure the reservations were reciprocated. But by the time we reached home, we were both certain that we were on the right track, and the foundation for a deep and special relationship was laid. Though we are both from different worlds, we found that mentally we could not have been more alike. Honestly, words are not quite sufficient to express our relationship. It was this rapport that helped us accomplish and strive for so much together, and it is the same feeling that brings Ken back to South India, again and again.

I mention this mainly to reassure those people who are dedicated to a cause. Perhaps there are others out there hoping to do good for people (humanity/less privilege). Where we come from is not the deciding factor—the individual is. Dr. Ken and his wife Eva have worked around the world from Africa to Indonesia, in refugee camps in Hong Kong, for the sake of children.

Both our families have become very close. We respect our differences and our cultural aim is to help those in need, no matter where they live. It has been my honor and privilege to have been able to become friends and associates with Ken and Eva Hobbs and their family. I sincerely wish and pray that there should be more like them in order to create more miracles.

Chennai (Madras) Rtn. PP. S.L. Chitale
Date: March 12, 1999

Foreword

My reasons for writing this story are very simple. For the first time in my life, I was brought face to face with the inequalities and injustices that children in the developing world must face. These inequalities are more than poverty or lack of food; their lives are not and have never been considered by the governments that rule them.

Secondly, I was exposed to the unproclaimed difference a committed organization, such as Rotary International, can and does make to eliminate these inequalities and injustices in the developing world.

I felt that this story of the introduction of measles vaccine into India in 1979 must be told. Not only to my fellow Rotarians but to the world in general. It is interesting to note that perhaps even the members of the Canadian committee will learn something of how and why the project was established. Obviously one cannot understand the magnitude and intricacies of the project when one visits the country on only two occasions over a fourteen-year period, for a total of five weeks on-site in the country.

This story could not have been told if there had not been a Rotarian by the name of Krish Chitale. Krish was the catalyst in India, as I was in Canada. Our chemistries met and produced an understanding and working relationship that has lasted over twenty-one years. His decisiveness and commitment to the poor in India is, indeed, an inspiration to all who have known him. This story will reveal his intense interest in the lives of the underprivileged in India.

To those who also played an important role in this miracle and who have not been mentioned personally by name, I apologize. It is an oversight rather than a deliberate omission. Without your help, the story would have never unfolded. This miracle is due to the committed Rotarians and government agencies, and in particular the District Collectors in the states of Tamil Nadu and Kearla.

Dr. Hande, the Minister of Health for the State of Tamil Nadu, was the catalyst in securing governmental co-operation with the Rotarian Red Measles Committee, chaired by Rotarian Krish Chitale.

Eva and I thank all of the Rotarians of South India and their wives for their kind hospitality and the understanding they afforded us. You were the reason for the miracle. You will always be able to tell your story to the future generations of South India, of the importance of this project by Rotary International, aided by the financial help of the Canadian government through it's International Development Agency.

I wish to thank my editor Doris Cowan for her help and suggestions, which are much appreciated. Thanks also to Gail Baird of Baird, O'Keefe Publishing Inc. for her personal help and suggestions.

Chapter 1

I know that miracles still happen. How do I know? Because I have experienced the magic: I have seen how miracles are made, and the influence some people can have in their creation.

The first miracle was the one that we all experience, but none of us can remember—my birth. My parents were loving, honest Christian people who believed that the world was as God made it, and that black was black and white was white and never the twain would meet. My father was a staunch believer in the Ten Commandments, and his faith in God never wavered. He was a conscientious civil servant, and a veteran of the First World War, who had been seriously wounded at Vimy Ridge. His injuries had necessitated the amputation of his lower right leg, as well as his left ring finger; he had also received multiple shrapnel wounds in his lower back. When the Depression struck, two years after my birth, my parents did their part. No one who came to our door asking for food was ever sent away hungry. Every Sunday we went to church, and I went to Sunday school. School was my most important responsibility, and there was never any question that I would accept it.

There were passages of rebellion, though, in the story of my growing up. One such period found me in the eastern Arctic. The year was 1945, and I was sixteen years old. It was a beautiful July morning and the sun was shining over the ice fields as the RMS *Nascopie* moved slowly forward. The *Nascopie* was a Hudson Bay supply ship that moved the RCMP officers to their various outposts and replenished their stores. I had signed on as a crew member for the four-month voyage, with my parents' reluctantly given permission, and I would not be home until October. School, I agreed, was important, but I knew I could miss a month or two without hurting my academic prospects. I could catch up.

And so it was that on that bright summer morning, far from home, the next miracle of my life occurred. As I looked out over the ice from the deck of the *Nascopie*, I experienced something like a sudden flash of light before my eyes, and I was gripped by the sudden compelling knowledge that I had to become a doctor. My life's purpose had opened before me, and my journey toward fulfilling my dream began at that moment. Sometimes I would be waylaid, or distracted from my goal, and the way forward was not to be without strife and turmoil, but never did I encounter an impasse or a dead end.

The next day I wrote to my mother. I told her of my decision to become a doctor, and recounted the sudden, inexplicable experience that had inspired my new ambition.

Her reaction was not enthusiastic. Knowing me as she did—remembering all too well the way I had resisted medical treatment in the past—she wondered if I was really suited to the medical profession. Over the next few months, after my return from the Arctic, she often asked me if I was still thinking the same way. She advised me to reconsider my decision, and forget the strange vision I had experienced that bright morning. I knew I would never forget it, but I also knew what she wanted to hear, and I reassured her, telling her that I would think it over carefully.

I date my lifelong belief in miracles from that episode.

The next few years brought stress and excitement. I still felt the pull of wanderlust. My love of travel was a compulsion, and June 1946 found me signing on as a crew member on the *Maria G.*, a tramp steamer of some 10,000 tons that had been built as a fort ship during the war. She was to be loaded with newsprint, and to depart from Montreal for Buenos Aires, via North Sydney and Botwood, Newfoundland. We arrived in Argentina in early September. My conscience told me that I should be starting school in Canada, but when our cargo was unloaded, we were filled with grain to carry to Antwerp in Belgium, and we did not get back to Saint John, New Brunswick, until December 19. My career as a sailor might have continued: when a sailor signs off and receives his pay at the purser's table, the captain sits at the next table and attempts to sign him up for the next trip before he leaves the ship. The *Maria G.* was about to set out on a seven-month, round-the world voyage that would not have seen me back in Canada again until the summer of 1947. I was tempted, but the strong inner commitment I had formed in 1945 stood me in good stead. My heart told me that another nine months out of school didn't matter—that it could make no difference one way or another— why not seize this chance to travel all around the world? Fortunately the voice of reason spoke to me: my inner voice said, not on your life, and I signed off and headed home for Christmas.

On January 3, 1947, I returned to high school. The next six months were stimulating—and rewarding—as I was able to complete five Grade 13 subjects with a very respectable average. I finished Grade 13 the next year with another five subjects. In September 1948, I entered pre-medicine at the University of Western Ontario, along with four hundred other hopefuls. University life was extremely enjoyable, yet I could not help wondering whether I would ever achieve my goal and graduate in medicine. I was only one among four hundred scholars and we could not all succeed.

After two years, only fifteen were accepted into medicine; unfortunately I was not one of the fifteen. I went on and received my BA (General Science) the following year. I was then accepted into the Faculty of Medicine.

In 1951, I began my medical studies, four years filled with hard work, excitement and new friendships. I have always maintained that the best years of my life were those I spent at university, and I would return today (if it were not for the obligation to write exams). I spent the summers as a cook on federal government topographic survey parties. These were small (five-man) groups, and working with them gave me a chance to do what I liked best: travel and explore. I worked in the Chibougamo area of Quebec, the interior of British Columbia, a hundred or so miles west of Williams Lake, and the mountains of the Yukon, both north and west of the settlement of Mayo. For the last two years of my medical studies, I lived at home with my parents in Ottawa. Once again I had the experience of being an at-home person, after several years on my own and being only a visitor to my family's house.

The most significant event of my life was my meeting with Eva Stumpf. Eva's parents had immigrated to Canada from Hungary; her father came in 1927 and her mother and two sisters joined him in 1929. Eighteen months later, Eva was born in Kitchener, Ontario. Her Hungarian sense of humor has been a real asset to me and to every person who has the privilege of knowing her. We fell in love, and were married on October 9, 1954, during my final year in medical school. She has been my strength. Whatever I have accomplished or attained I owe to her. She has been my confidante, and the mother of our three children; she has been cook, *dobbie* (laundry) lady, secretary, and companion to me wherever in this good world we have lived and traveled.

In May of 1954, I was back at my regular Ottawa summer job, working for the local bakery, Morrison Lamothe. My last exam had been written a month before, and one morning I was delivering bread to a grocery store on Preston Street, in the Italian section of town. When I walked in, the owner greeted me with, "Mr. Baker, I mean Mr. Doctor, your father wants you to phone him." At that moment I knew that my ten-year dream had come true. I received my MD on June 4, 1955.

My year as an intern was long, difficult, tiring, and frustrating. The Ottawa Civic Hospital paid me $90 a month, minus $10 for room and board. I was on call every other night and every other weekend. In May of that year, I decided to seek a residency in general practice at the Ohio Valley General Hospital in Wheeling, West Virginia. I was accepted, and Eva and I, feeling rich and secure on my salary of $300 a month, moved to Wheeling and began a new life. On Easter Sunday, April 21, 1957, our first-born, John, came into the world. The other important event of those years was the beginning of my friendship with my future medical partner, George Jaciw. George, too, was a Canadian. He had immigrated to

Canada from the Ukraine in 1947, following the war. His immense desire and ambition allowed him to pass through very difficult times and graduate from the University of Ottawa with an MD in 1955. He had interned at the Ottawa General Hospital and was in Wheeling doing a year of general surgery. We discovered a mutual affinity, and before the year was out we had decided to enter general practice together. His charming wife, Martha, became a close friend as well, and our friendship has lasted over these forty years.

George and I started up our practice in Whitby, Ontario, in July 1957. The next few years were busy ones for Eva and me, full of happy new experiences and the odd frustration. Our first daughter, Anne Elizabeth, was born on April 19, 1958; on April 11, 1960, she was followed by Mary Katherine, and our family was complete.

I soon became actively involved with the community, beginning with the public school board. I was first elected to the board in 1959, and served as its chairman from 1960 to 1965. I then decided that I would venture a little farther into politics, and ran for mayor. I was soundly defeated. The winner was Desmond Newman, whom I later came to know well, and to respect and admire (in spite of having lost the election to him); he is a good friend. Desmond was mayor until 1973, and no leader in any community that I know of has left a more positive record. I joined him as an elected councilor in 1967, and served in that capacity until 1976. (In 1976 I again ran for high office, and was once again defeated.)

Whitby was very much in need of a general hospital, and I became active in the drive to create one. I was appointed to the steering committee in 1959, acted as site committee chairman and was elected to the board of governors in 1962, then went on to become chairman of the building committee, chairman of the board, and finally chief of staff. In 1981, I decided that after twelve years of working for the hospital I had contributed all that I could, and that it was time for other people to step forward.

My wanderlust was still with me. In 1964, Eva and I bought a 25-foot travel trailer. Over the next fifteen years we explored every province and almost all of the continental forty-nine states. We spent a minimum of six weeks travelling the USA and Canada every year.

During my early years of medical practice, I was introduced to the concept of the service club. I was asked to be a charter member of the local Lions' Club in 1959, but it wasn't long before I decided that Lionism was not for me. I was appointed "Tail Twister," and during the first governor's visit, I cut off his tie when he refused to sing. I had not anticipated that a grown man would cry over the loss of his tie. Justifiably or not, his wife became rude and insulting. Thus ended my career as a Lion.

The next service club that I tried was the Kiwanis. It was 1967, the year of centennial celebrations, and I felt that I should try to contribute more. I had been invited to join the Kiwanis Club, and I decided to accept. It was very different from the Lions and for a while I enjoyed the comradeship—especially the annual fishing trips. However, as a municipal councilor, I had meetings practically every evening, Monday through Friday. Setting aside Thursday evenings for club meetings was difficult, and in any case it seemed to me that they were becoming an excuse for a night out drinking. I was never a teetotaler, then or now, but I did conclude that I was not getting what I had expected out of a service club. I began to resent spending a night away from Eva and the family. After four years with the Kiwanis, I decided to resign my membership, and I vowed that never again would I join a service club, no matter what.

However!

On the first Tuesday of May, 1976, my dear friend Bill Nurse invited me to be his guest at the Rotary Club. As the president, he told me, he had made a commitment to bring in five new members during his year, and his year ended on June 30. He hoped that I would consent to join the club temporarily. He assured me that he would reimburse me double the money I had laid out if I decided to leave after July 1.

I tried to explain that I had decided that I would never join another service club, that as far as such organizations were concerned I was a two-time loser, and that I was definitely not interested. But at the back of my mind, as I made my excuses, I found myself remembering all the support Bill had given me on the hospital board, and what he had promised to do for me in the upcoming election for mayor. Suddenly, much to my surprise, I heard myself agreeing to accompany him to Rotary.

The Rotary luncheon Bill took me to turned out to be another turning point. It introduced me to the true meaning of what a service club can and should do.

Chapter 2

I was now a Rotarian. I was inducted into the club in the middle of May 1976. At first I was not entirely comfortable with my decision. However, I had known most of the eighty-five members for a number of years, through either my medical practice or my political activities. During my work with the committees that were struck to found the Whitby General Hospital, I had come to know some members very well. They were good friends, and I kept my doubts to myself. But I was still not convinced of the value of any service club, not even Rotary.

The first of July came along and I was still attending meetings, even though my friend Bill Nurse was no longer president. The Rotary year had ended (it runs from the first of July until the end of June the following year) and it was time for me to make a definite decision. The membership let me know that if I was to experience the true meaning of fellowship in Rotary, I would have to delve a little deeper into the club's background. They offered to instruct me.

Over the weeks of my introduction to the principles of the organization, I slowly became convinced that the Rotary had an integrity that I had not found in the other two service clubs I had tried. (As I look back on it now, I suspect that it was not the fault of the Lions or the Kiwanis that I had found them wanting, but my own. When I was younger I was simply not ready to accept the responsibilities that membership entailed.) I was impressed with what I was now learning about Rotary's aims and ideals.

The most persuasive part of their message was the "four way test," which is the true heart of the Rotary movement. Before embarking on

· 1976 – 1979 ·

any venture or making any decision or statement, a Rotarian is required to ask himself four questions: 1) Is it the truth? 2) Is it fair to all concerned? 3) Will it build good will and better friendships? 4) Will it be beneficial to all concerned? I was also impressed by the club's motto: "Service above Self" and "He profits most who serves best."

I knew that if I made a decision to continue in Rotary, I would have to become more significantly involved, and more knowledgeable of the principles and organizational structure of Rotary. In May 1978, I attended a District Assembly and my appetite was whetted. All I knew at this point was that Rotary had been the first service club in the world. It was founded in Chicago by Paul Harris, a lawyer; Sylvester Schell, a coal dealer; Gus Loehr, a mining engineer; and Hiram Shorey, a merchant tailor. In 1910, when a club was chartered in Winnipeg, Rotary had become international. (It is now established in more countries and geographical areas than there are in the United Nations.)

Rotary offers four avenues of service through which a member can choose to make a contribution: Club Service, Community Service, Vocational Service, and International Service. I began to realize why we had a classification system regarding new members. It made sense. Since the beginning, Paul Harris had stressed that no more than two members of a club could belong to the same profession or avocation. This rule meant that each club was a cross-section of the community. If membership had been left to chance, many clubs would have been composed of only one or two professions or avocations. The diversity and strength of Rotary is in this simple classification principle; it is not found in any other service club organization.

Eva and I soon made a major step in becoming a committed Rotarian family: we offered to host our club's first exchange student. Julie arrived from Australia in January 1978 and stayed with us for more than five months. She was the first of nine students that we would host over the next eight years.

In January 1979, we took our second step. I attended a district zone meeting. This was a large gathering, the main purpose of which was to bring the Rotarians over a large area up to date on what was happening within the district. In 1979, there were approximately 450 districts in the world. Ours was District 707; it encompassed sixty-eight clubs, from Guelph in the west, to Belleville in the east, and as far north as Alliston.

At the social time before lunch, Joe Southwell, a member of our club, bought me a Scotch. Joe and I had been friends for several years. He was the chairman of the World Community Service Committee for the district, and I was glad to have a chance to talk to him about possible ways I could contribute to the work of the committee. I had more than once expressed to medical colleagues my interest in the possibility of working, on a short-term basis, in troubled parts of the developing world. I had thought of the church, but I felt that this might put restrictions on me. I have never been a person who wears religion on his sleeve. My religious commitments have always been very personal, private and individualistic.

Now, at lunch, I told Joe Southwell about my interest in the developing world and asked him about the work of the World Community Service Committee. He was very pleased that I was interested in lending a hand. There were several projects on the go in the district at the time, he told me. One was a project in Haiti, called "Heifers to Haiti." They were shipping a load of heifers, via Air Canada, on a cargo flight in two or three weeks' time. He asked if I would like to come down to the airport and see the cattle off. He also suggested that, if I was interested, I would be most welcome to accompany the committee to Haiti three weeks after the shipment, at my own expense, of course. I told him that it sounded very exciting, and immediately agreed to go.

Over dessert, the conversation turned to a letter that had recently been sent out to all members of District 707 by Governor Bud Crookes (every Rotary district has an elected governor who acts as CEO for one year). In the letter, Governor Crookes had proposed an International Service program to supply measles, mumps and rubella (German measles) vaccines in South India. I told Joe that I would like to talk with the governor. I knew that the program would be very expensive, and I personally felt that vaccination against measles was by far the most important. Measles, I explained to Joe, kills more children than any other disease that can be prevented by immunization. Joe sounded very encouraged that I had at last made a commitment to become involved. He told me that after the cattle were shipped, we would talk with Governor Bud Crookes.

The day the cattle were to be flown to Haiti was a beautiful February morning. Joe picked me up and we headed for the airport. Their scheduled departure time was 12:30 p.m., and Joe had promised me that I would be back in my office by 3:30 p.m. Plans, plans, plans! What fools they make of us. The plane did not leave at 12:30, but rather at 4:30 p.m.—the authorities in Port-au-Prince were making difficulties about our permission to land. Time was growing short, and there were no lights on the airfield in Port-au-Prince; the cattle had been loaded and waiting on the plane for some two and a half hours. Finally, after lengthy negotiations, they were given permission to land, and the Air Canada cargo plane departed.

As we left the airport, I had the opportunity of a brief conversation with Governor Bud. I expressed my interest in the India project, and explained my views on the appropriateness of emphasizing the measles vaccine over the others. He understood and agreed with my concerns, and asked if I would take on the job of delivering the vaccine to India. I knew that the budget for the trip was not large and I offered to go on condition that I personally paid all of Eva's and my expenses and airfares, as I did not want any of measles project money to be spent on anything but the project itself. Governor Bud and I agreed that we would discuss the trip in more detail when we were in Haiti in three weeks' time.

The early seeds of the miracle had been planted!

Chapter 3

We met at the Toronto International Airport on the morning of March 20, 1979. In the group were the present district governor, Bud Crookes, the incoming governor, Paul McKelvey; Joe Southwell and Bill Irwin from my club; three other Rotarians from the district, and myself. We flew to Dorval Airport in Montreal, then changed planes and headed for Port-au-Prince. As I recall, we arrived in Port-au-Prince in early afternoon. A dirty old DC3 was at our disposal to carry us the 125 miles to Les Cayes at the southern tip of the island. The plane was the "Air Force One" belonging to the president of the country, Jean-Claude Duvalier (better known as "Baby Doc," after his father "Papa Doc," who was "president-for-life" before him). Before our departure, we were served a bite to eat and drinks. The Les Cayes Rotarians met us on our arrival, and we had an enjoyable evening of fellowship.

We stayed that night in Les Cayes. The accommodations were not what I was used to! However, over the next sixteen years of Rotary travel, I was often to remind myself that, in comparison with the conditions that local people had to put up with, this was like staying at the Ritz.

The following day we flew back to Port-au-Prince and stayed the night in a very posh hotel on the side of the hill overlooking the city of Port-au-Prince. Next morning, accompanied by armed escorts, we headed by bus to Cape Haitian, one hundred miles to the north, at the top end of the island. Here the true meaning of our project was brought home to me when I saw, first-hand, milk from our Rotary cows being given to a group of hungry, underprivileged children. These were orphans who were cared for by a Dutch order of priests. Seeing them, I began to wonder how many Canadian heifers had ended up on Baby Doc's barbecue.

On our return to Port-au-Prince we visited a school and in the evening were entertained by local Rotarians and their wives. The affluence of these influential people, in such a poor environment, still stands out in my memory.

Finally, on our flight home, I had a meeting with Governor Bud and DGN (district governor nominee) Paul McKelvey.

Our discussions were brief and to the point. The decision was made that I would take the measles vaccine to India in early September 1979. I was left with the impression that everything was in order, and all I had to do was buy our tickets and we would be off to India in early September. How wrong I was!

In April I received a notice that I was invited to attend the District World Community Service meeting, on April 28 at the Purina Feed Company's boardroom in Whitby. The invitation included an agenda for the meeting. The last item was under new business: "Ken Hobbs and the measles project with Rotary Club of Madras."

I arrived at the appointed time, eager to learn what the next steps would be. Methodically, the committee went through the agenda. When we reached the Hobbs-Madras item, the chairman turned to me and asked for my report on what I had done, what the budget was, how we were going to raise the funds, etc. With a shock I realized that it was all up to me—I was both the chairman and the committee of one. I had to explain that almost nothing had been done.

On my way home after the meeting I contemplated how I could proceed with this project. I had volunteered, but I had not realized that very little in the way of concrete planning had been done by anyone. Nothing was on paper except the hopes of two district governors who had met almost a year ago, in Boca Raton, Florida, during their training session. They had proposed that an MMR (measles, mumps, and rubella) immunization should be carried out between their two districts in celebration of the International Year of the Child. One of the two was Governor Bud Crookes of District 707; the other was Governor P. Jagatheesan of District 320, which takes in most of the state of Kerala and all of the state of Tamil Nadu in southern India.

Governor Bud had forwarded the history of the project to me. It consisted of a brief exchange of letters and notes; it was scanty, but a place to start. On 14 December 1978, Governor Bud had written Dr. Ralph Henderson of the World Health Organization (WHO) in Geneva, and he had received an answer. In his reply, dated December 20, 1978, Dr. Henderson gave some specific suggestions about consulting with the WHO office in New Delhi. He also expressed his appreciation of Rotary's willingness to get involved in immunization. He wrote: " We have just received your letter, a few days before Christmas, and I can't think of a more welcome tiding for our program."

On January 1, 1979, Governor Bud wrote to his counterpart, Governor P. Jagatheesan of District 320. He informed him that our district was in a go position after receiving the letter from Dr. Henderson of WHO, Geneva, Switzerland, and that he had asked a member of his club, Dr. Rostogi, to correspond with MSD (Merck, Sharpe and Dohme, an American pharmaceutical firm with a Canadian subsidiary in Montreal, manufacturers of drugs and vaccines) regarding MMR vaccine. Governor P.J. replied, stating that he was asking a past president of the Rotary Club of Madras, R.P. Sarathy, to reply to him separately regarding the number of doses of measles vaccine that they required. This letter, dated January 12, specifically states "measles vaccine," and not MMR. No letter to Governor Bud from Past President Sarathy ever materialized. On 8 May 1979, Bud wrote to Mr. Sarathy, noting that he has not had any response from him, and indicating that Governor P.J.'s letter of January 12 had led him to expect some communication. He goes on to tell Rotarian Sarathy that a Canadian delegate (myself) would be arriving, before the vaccine, in September; and that perhaps he could arrange accommodation for me and my wife during my stay. He further notes that Dr. Rostogi would be visiting Madras in June and would like to have a meeting with his committee to work out the final details.

In my mind the project was established and ready to go, but from the evidence of the letters, or rather the lack of letters, before me, I now realized that there were several threads still loose and the only person who could collect them and tie them was myself. First, I had to solve the problem of whether we were sending MMR or red measles vaccine (rubeola). Governor Bud had left that up to me and I accepted his endorsement. Over the first several days in May 1979, I was in communication via telephone with Merck, Sharpe and Dohme in their Montreal office. I talked to Mr. Landry, the district sales manager, and Mr. Lee, the manager of pricing services. On May 9, 1979, Mr. Landry forwarded me the conditions of MSD's shipment of MMR to Madras. However, Mr. Lee's letter of May 15 gave the price of Attenuvax, the vaccine for red measles alone, at 25 cents US per dose, including diluent, in 10-millilitre vials; the method of payment would be by irrevocable confirmed letter of credit. I would be responsible for securing all approvals to allow the vaccine into India, and the freight charges would be the responsibility of Rotary. They further stated that they would be able to supply up to 100,000 doses by 15 September 1979.

The Toronto Don Mills Rotary club applied to CIDA (the Canadian International Development Agency) on 17 May 1979 for a grant of $32,250 (Cdn). The Rotary clubs of District 707 had agreed to contribute $6,750, and Rotary International $4,000, for a combined budget of $43,000 (Cdn.), which would supply 120,000 doses of live red measles vaccine. I was now confident that the trials and tribulations were over.

Or were they just beginning?

The immediate problems were twofold; first, I had to secure approval for the vaccine to enter India; second, I had to somehow arrange free air transport of the vaccine from New York to Madras. I contacted Dr. Rostogi and asked his opinion as to how I could go about resolving these two issues. He suggested that we meet with Mr. Soni, the Indian trade commissioner in Toronto.

On May 24, we met with Mr. Soni at his residence. Unfortunately, he was not helpful. He expressed his approval, but he went on to state very firmly that there was nothing he or the Indian High Commissioner in Ottawa could do to offer any assistance in these two important matters. However, he did advise us that we would have to obtain the approval, in writing, of the Madras Ministry of Health and the federal Ministry of Health in New Delhi. Once I had these written endorsements, he would attempt to get the Indian High Commissioner in Ottawa to approve the free air shipment.

This meeting was the first of many I would have with Indian government officials over the next several years. I had always been accustomed to receiving direct answers to direct questions, clear statements of approval or disapproval—in other words, a straight yes or no. Now I was to learn what it was like to get both at the same time.

I decided that I would attempt to reach Governor P.J. directly, by telephoning Coimbatore. This was my first experience of the Indian telephone system—and what an experience it was. I first had to go through the Bell telephone operator in Montreal, who connected me with an operator in London, England, who in turn reached a Bombay operator, who rang the number in Coimbatore. With the intervention of each operator, the volume dropped lower and lower, and when P.J. finally came on the phone I could barely hear his voice, let alone understand what he was saying. However, in three weeks, I did receive from him a copy of a letter to Past President Sarathy in which he gave directions to the Rotary Club concerning the securing of official approval from the ministry of health. In Governor P.J.'s letter he also mentioned another Rotarian, Krish Chitale. This name was unknown to me then, but it was to become very familiar to me over the course of my adventures in India.

Governor Bud Crookes forwarded me a copy of a letter from Krish Chitale, dated 30 May 1979, giving all the pertinent details of the requirements for free clearance of the vaccine of customs duty charges. But we had still not received formal clearance of the vaccine from the state Ministry of Health. Chitale emphasized that the shipment must be addressed to "The Rotary Club of Madras, Charitable Trust."

On May 31, MSD confirmed the order for 13,808 ten-dose vials, plus diluent, of Attenuvax (red measles vaccine), at a price of $40,000 (Cdn), to be shipped from Kennedy Airport, with an estimated delivery date of September 15, 1979.

I thought that with everything now on stream, Eva and I could go ahead and book our flight. The year 1979 was an important milestone for us: it was our twenty-fifth wedding anniversary. We decided to take a trip around the world—a trip that would include a four- or five-week stay in the south of India.

In early June I received a telephone call from Mr. Barry O'Neill of CIDA. He was inquiring about our proposed red measles immunization project. The thought that the project might be approved for funding by CIDA rekindled my enthusiasm. However, getting final approval for it was an arduous task. I wrote to our member of Parliament, Mr. Scott Fennell (Conservative member for the riding of Durham South) in mid-July. He forwarded copies of our correspondence to Senator Asselin, the head of CIDA, together with statements of his own support for the project, on July 24. Approval was granted on August 20, 1979, for the sum of $34,400 (Cdn). The final financial peg was now in place.

On July 5, the Indian state ministry of health also gave us a positive response and Krish Chitale sent a "true copy" of their endorsement. However, this turned out not to be the same federal ministry of health whose endorsement would allow Mr. Soni and the Indian High Commissioner to authorize free air transport of the vaccine. I wrote Krish (Krish Chitale is a member of the Rotary Club of Madras; he is also the most outstanding architect of that city of 5.5 million. He was to become a good friend; hereinafter he will be referred to as Krish) on the first of August, outlining what was still required. I also enclosed our travel plans: our departure date from Canada and our expected arrival date in Madras. I was still very confident that all the bridges had now been crossed, and that the problems that remained to be solved were minor and insignificant.

MSD telephoned me on August 20, stating that they could only supply 68,000 doses of Attenuvax vaccine, and that these would be single-dose vials, and at the same cost as the 138,000 doses originally offered, which were in 10 cc vials. The change to a smaller amount was due to our requirement of a conditional order based on CIDA's approval of funding, and the international demand for measles vaccine.

Tuesday morning, August 27, was indeed memorable. The previous day, we had purchased our world-tour tickets, which were non-refundable, and we were making our final preparations for departure. I was in my office, and I was in for a shock.

My secretary informed me that CNCP telecommunications had a message for me. An agent was on the phone. He told me that a telegram from India had been received for me, and read out the following: "Government approval delayed by unexpected development at Delhi. Health Minister opinions that WHO approves only Schwarz strain of measles vaccine for tropics. Please confirm. Will advise progress early September and when it will be suitable for your visit and the shipment of the vaccine. Chitale."

I sat quietly, thunderstruck. What was I to do now? Hours later, still in a daze, I went to Rotary. I walked into the curling club, and Bill Nurse, seeing my dumbfounded expression, realized immediately that something was terribly wrong. I told him about the telegram I had received from Krish.

It appeared that this difficulty, fortunately, could be solved over the next twenty-four hours. When I awoke the next morning, August 28, I remembered that Bill Nurse had a telex in his Chev-Olds dealership. I knew that Bill would offer the use of it if I needed it—all I had to do was ask.

I contacted Mr. Lee of MSD in Montreal and explained the problem. Could he help us by supplying the essential facts? He was happy to be of assistance. The Schwartz measles virus vaccine, he noted, was an older type; the Edmonston strain was a modification of the Enders strain, which in turn had been a further attenuated strain of the Schwartz strain of measles virus. (A virus is attenuated by passing it through chick embryos, in order to produce a vaccine that has fewer side effects and elicits a more potent immunological response.) The war of Schwartz versus Edmonston would continue for the next several months. The bureaucracy in New Delhi were very resistant. They were relying on old scientific data and were reluctant to accept the newer, safer, more effective type of vaccine that was now being produced. The solution to this problem was now clear (I hoped). I remembered the letter that Governor Bud Crookes had written to Dr. Henderson of WHO in Geneva in December 1978. With the help of Bill Nurse, I drafted a telex and forwarded it to Dr. Henderson in Geneva that same day.

In the telex, I presented the Schwartz-versus-Edmonston problem and asked for his assistance in clearing up this misunderstanding with the Ministry of Health in New Delhi.

Dr. Henderson replied almost immediately. He asked us to request that MSD forward their criteria on their Edmonston strain of measles vaccine to him. Perhaps, he wrote, the New Delhi officials were confused because we would not be using the further attenuated Edmonston strain of vaccine. He also asked for the manufacturer's scientific stability data on the Attenuvax vaccine. This information was sent to Dr. Henderson on August 29. A telegram was also dispatched to Krish Chitale in Madras, informing him of my correspondence with WHO in Geneva. I stressed that the vaccine we were sending was not contraindicated in the tropics. I also related to Krish that we would be leaving Canada on September 5 and would arrive in Madras on September 14 at 8:35 p.m. on Indian Airlines, flight 171.

MSD were very co-operative in replying to all my requests for this important information. As we headed into the long Labour Day weekend, Bill Nurse insisted that I take the keys to his dealership in order to monitor the telex machine over the holiday. Dr. Henderson sent telexes to me on the 5th, 7th and 11th of September. His telex of the 11th was significant (even though I was already in India by the time it arrived). It read as follows:

> We are informed that drug controller Government of India has not yet approved Edmonston further attenuated strain of measles vaccine stop an urgent opinion being sought in response to your requests but this is an internal government process and approval of this vaccine by WHO does not oblige government to accept it stop we continue to hope this will be resolved satisfactorily stop. Henderson, UNISANTE, Geneva.

On September 14, Bill Nurse sent a telex to me in Madras, stating that he had received a telegram from Krish Chitale with the news that the Indian government had approved the vaccine. Governor Bud Crookes was awaiting my reply before confirming the final details of the shipment of vaccine from New York. I sent a reply after arriving in Madras on Saturday, September 15.

Twenty-eight telexes would be sent and received by the Nurse Chevrolet Oldsmobile dealership over the next four months.

Chapter 4

Wednesday, September 5 arrived. I tried to put my worries out of my mind, but just below the surface of my consciousness doubts disturbed me; I wondered if the project could possibly succeed. As we packed, Eva and I discussed the itinerary of our three-month round-the-world pilgrimage. Our travel agent had told us that we could check in three bags each, plus a carry-on. We believed her, of course—much to our later dismay.

Eva packed one suitcase full of eatables: cookies, granola bars, candies, tea bags and soda crackers. Someone had told her that India was very short of food and that we had better be prepared. We packed all types of clothing—for wet, dry, cold, warm, and hot weather. I had assembled a variety of antibiotics, sterile dressings, chloroquin (our anti-malarial medication), etc. In one suitcase, I packed the automatic injection immunization gun along with its CO_2 tank. We thought we were ready for any unexpected eventuality.

However, we didn't expected what happened next.

At 12:20 p.m., five hours before we were to leave, the phone rang. It was our travel agent. Air India, she told us, was on strike out of London; we would have to make alternative arrangements with Alitalia Airlines in London for our flight to Rome. She had booked us on Air Canada from Toronto to New York; Air India from New York to London; and now Alitalia from London to Rome. Then we would be back on schedule in Rome with Air India to Bombay. This appeared to be a minor inconvenience, but it was just a foreshadowing of the many we would experience over the next three months.

Diary of a Miracle

Joe Southwell and his wife, Helen, arrived at 5:30 p.m. sharp to take us to the Toronto International Airport. For Joe to be on time was a miracle in itself: I took it as an omen that other miracles would surely be created on our expedition. Helen remarked on Eva's white straw hat, which resembled those worn by the ladies of the Salvation Army; I soon christened it her "missionary hat." For the next two weeks, Eva was either wearing it or carrying it in her hand. I tried, but failed, to persuade her to leave it behind or pack it in one of the six suitcases we were carrying.

Our flight to New York was uneventful. We were riding high on adrenaline, with great expectations of our leap into the unknown. We knew we would encounter stark cultural differences in South India, but whether they would be enjoyable, or the reverse of enjoyable, we had no idea.

The flight out of New York on Air India was delayed, but eventually we were on our way. The cultural differences began immediately. We were asked whether we wanted "veggie or non veggie" (vegetarian or meat curry) for our dinner. Our meal was uninteresting and spicy hot, which bothered Eva. The stewardesses were dressed in saris; a good percentage of the passengers were Indian, and Eva and I were amazed and fascinated by their style of dress.

We arrived in London at 11:00 a.m. local time, and after making inquiries at the Air India desk, we sought out a taxi to take us to the Cumberland Hotel.

The Cumberland was centrally located, close to Hyde Park; the main shopping district was only a short walk away. After checking in at the hotel, we decided that we had better reconfirm our tickets on Alitalia Airlines for our flight to Rome on Sunday, September 9. On presenting our tickets to Alitalia, we discovered that Air India in Toronto had not prearranged our flight from London to Rome. A visit to the Air Canada office soon solved our problems with the tickets. Our reservations were confirmed. We were scheduled to leave on the Sunday morning flight to Rome.

· September 1979 ·

The next two days were spent sightseeing in London: Westminster Abbey, London Bridge, lunch at the Post Office tower, excursions on the double-decker buses. At the end of a hectic forty-eight hours, we were ready for another new experience: Rome.

Our flight to Rome was uneventful, but on our arrival, I was shocked to see so many armed military personnel in the airport, with submachine guns slung casually over their shoulders. I have never liked guns of any type—high-powered, low-powered or multiple automatic, I am equally unenthusiastic about them all. Our taxi ride to the hotel was stimulating in yet another way. Our driver acted as if he was on the Grand Prix circuit. After many narrow escapes we arrived at the hotel.

Our room at the charming old Bernini Bristol Hotel was very elegant and impressive. After reading the instructions on how to use the phone, I decided it would be easier to forget about it. Our room overlooked the entrance to the hotel, and had a small balcony, ideally placed to watch the river of life swirling past in the street. The traffic was extremely interesting to watch; I wondered why there were not more accidents. No driver ever gave way until the last second. The beautiful, bra-less young Italian women were a delight to gaze upon, to say the least. The rest of the day was spent at an outdoor sidewalk cafe, admiring the scenery.

After breakfast on Monday, we called the Air India office to verify our flight from Rome to Bombay. They informed us that our tickets were scheduled for August, not September. However, they could accommodate us on the evening flight on Wednesday, September 12. We had been scheduled to leave on Thursday, September 13, or so we had been told. I started to wonder whether it was our travel agent or Air India that was confused. Later, I realized that Indian bureaucracy, whether it was the government or a private corporation, was at the best of times completely disorganized.

We spent the rest of Monday doing "tourist" things in Rome.

On Tuesday we decided to take an all-day trip to Salerno and the Isle of Capri. The trip was exhausting. However, the beauty of the Blue

Grotto and the surrounding countryside made up for exhaustion. We returned to Rome late in the evening.

On Wednesday morning we toured the Vatican, where we learned about the long, impressive history of this most influential enclave, which has given so much to the world. The afternoon was spent repacking and preparing ourselves for the unpredictable adventures that lay ahead of us. At checkout, the manager attempted to charge me for our rooms, which had been prepaid. Fortunately I had the receipts with me, and he had to back down. However, he then presented me with a telephone bill for the equivalent of $250 (US). When I refused to pay the charges he became belligerent. I attempted to explain to him that I had never picked up the phone, and the conversation became even louder. Finally his supervisor appeared from the inner sanctum. I pointed out that the calls had been made by room 214, and that we were in room 212. In a few minutes the problem was solved.

At the airport our baggage was X-rayed, and the check-in person became very upset and confronted us, ordering me to open one of our suitcases, the one that contained the empty CO_2 tank. This was part of the Medijet immunization gun that I was taking to India. It uses CO_2 as an expellant, and I have to admit that on the X-ray it did resemble a bomb. After a lot of difficulty, I found the key to the suitcase, and was able to prove to him that it was innocuous. Interesting that our suitcases had been X-rayed in Toronto, New York and London, and this was the first time that anyone had questioned the bomb-like device in our luggage!

We boarded the giant 747 and I was perplexed to find that there were only about forty-five passengers in evidence. Our seats were in the tail section. After a few minutes the captain's voice came on the intercom, announcing that there would be a significant delay in our departure. Cocktails and supper would be served, but our scheduled departure time, 9:45, was changed to sometime after 11:30 p.m.

While we were having our drinks, a small, insignificant-looking man came in, carrying a long and fairly large leather case, which he placed opposite the empty center aisle seats. He was soon greeted warmly by most of the stewardesses. I said to Eva that he must be a VIP, but why would a VIP be sitting in economy? Throughout our flight I kept pondering the mystery. Who was he, and why was he sitting in economy on a jet plane that would normally carry some four hundred passengers, but on this flight was carrying no more than fifty?

After supper, I moved to the center rows, put the arm supports down, and immediately fell asleep. The night hours passed swiftly. At breakfast time I went back to my regular seat, and resumed my observation of the continuous flow of stewardesses to the mystery person in the seat ahead of us. We landed in Bombay at 10:45 a.m. on Thursday, September 13. As the plane touched down, the very short mystery gentleman turned to me and asked, "Is this your first visit to my country?"

"Yes," I replied.

"I am Ravi Shankar," he then informed me, "and I always travel Air India because they are the only airline in the world that allows me to keep my instrument on the plane with me." Ravi Shankar is the world's most famous performer on the sitar, a long-necked instrument with unique melodic and drone strings capable of creating extremely haunting and beautiful music. Shankar had taught the Beatles to play and chord their guitars in the Indian style, and George Harrison to play the sitar, and here he was, welcoming us to India. "I know that you will enjoy and love my country," he said to us, "if you take time to appreciate our culture and differences."

This was perhaps the most sincere and positive welcome anybody could have to the mysterious subcontinent of India.

Chapter 5

As we stepped out of the giant Air India 747, we were hit with a wave of warmth, humidity, noise, and smells. For a moment we stood aghast—we had really landed in this historic city of Bombay.

We became aware that we were being signaled to by a short, stout Indian soldier, who despite the heat was dressed in a very heavy, winter-issue khaki uniform, complete with shorts. He wore a heavy tunic, puttees, heavy boots, and a recognizable Bengal-Lancer hat; all this even though the outside temperature was almost 40 degrees Celsius, with a humidity reading of almost 95 percent. He looked like a young man, but on closer examination I could see that his face was weather-beaten and the wide handlebar mustache he sported was graying. He was calling, "No! no! sir—you must come this way." His accent made him almost impossible to understand. Eva quickly said, "I think we are going in the wrong direction." We turned and approached the guard who pointed to the pile of baggage on the tarmac, at the same time scrutinizing us closely. "When you have your baggage, sir, you must bring it to me for initial inspection before entering the reception hall."

It became obvious that we would have to carry our own baggage, all six pieces including our carry-ons. When we finally had carried the luggage up the six or so steps, the guard methodically marked each piece of our luggage with a yellow piece of chalk, then handed me six small pieces of paper, with curious figures inscribed on them. We decided that Eva would go inside the hall and get in line and I would make a couple of trips with the luggage.

Perspiration was flowing off my face, hands, and chest like a turned-on water faucet. Finally we cleared immigration and headed for the customs check. Unfortunately, one of the chalk marks, on the largest bag, had rubbed off against my pants as I carried it. In a harsh, officious voice, the customs agent announced, "This bag has not been properly cleared, please attend to it."

I had to retrace my steps to the guard outside to have another chalk mark put on the bag. I was given another piece of paper with the same curious markings, which as far as I could see were of no significance.

Ten minutes later, when I arrived back at the customs desk, Eva appeared to be in a trance. She was staring up across the room toward the window some ten feet from where she was standing. All you could see, pressed against the dirty glass, were the faces of children, one piled on top of the other, appearing to go right to the ceiling. We stood for a moment staring with sheer amazement.

The customs official directed us to open our bags. I started with the smallest, figuring that he would be satisfied with examining one; that, however, was not to be. Thirty minutes later we were given permission to repack all of our luggage and leave.

Once outside the reception hall, we were greeted by all the faces that had been stacked against the window. A sea of hands held out their dirty palms, begging faces were turned to us, faces with dirty runny noses, phlegm which ran down their upper lips and blemished cheeks. Their clothes were tattered and their feet were bare, but they were all smiling, displaying white teeth that absolutely glistened in the bright sunlight, reminding me of the advertisements for Close-up toothpaste. Then came the onslaught of baggage handlers, all attempting to grab your bags and disappear with them to their favorite taxi drivers, who were obviously in cahoots with them. Absolute bedlam! I was not able to take charge of the situation; I was being manipulated by a bunch of taxi drivers and baggage handlers. The pestering appeals of the children added to the disorganization and impossible confusion. Their tiny dirty hands were stretched out towards us—as you looked down all you could see were hands, and the older teenagers were trying to grab our luggage. Finally I became annoyed and halted the process with a sudden exclamation, choosing a baggage handler and a taxi driver at random. Eva got into the cab, while I attempted to supervise the loading of the luggage into the trunk of the taxi. This was no mean feat: as soon as I suggested a method, the bearers of the luggage and the taxi driver disagreed vehemently. After much frustration I made sure that the luggage would not fall out of the trunk and everything was in order.

Soaked in sweat, I climbed into the small taxi. It was clear that the trip to the Taj Mahal Hotel was going to be an experience the like of which we had never had. No sooner were we out of the airport than the reality of culture shock hit home. We had expected a large city. Bombay is the capital of the western Indian state of Maharastra; it is the largest metropolis in the country, with two-thirds of the population concentrated on Bombay Island. We knew, too, that Bombay has one of the highest population densities in the world (1,500 per square mile). But for the next hour we were assailed by sights that we never dreamed of. The road was lined with the homes of the untouchables of Bombay. All along the main road into the city were hovels made of cardboard, metal panels, scraps of wood, shacks placed right at the curb: for miles they were all you could see.

The traffic was unbelievable. Cars, trucks, buses, bullock carts, bicycles, three wheelers (motorized bicycles used as taxis by the poorer people), pedestrians, and, every now and then, cattle. Cows were roaming freely through the traffic; some cows were lying down, tired, in the middle of the road for a lengthy rest, while motorcycles whizzed around them carrying everything and everybody including up to three extra passengers. Mothers rode sidesaddle in their beautiful saris, some holding more than one infant. Our taxi was completely surrounded by vehicles and people, walking or pushing carts laden with goods, produce or animals. This went on for the entire length of our journey to the Taj Hotel. As we approached the center of the city the traffic became even heavier. The concentration of people, vehicles and

Bombay, September 1979

animals was simply astounding. We looked at each other in amazement, unable to speak, dumbfounded by what we were witnessing.

Then our taxi pulled into the entranceway of the Taj Hotel, and we were greeted by a tall, sophisticated-looking doorman, dressed in typical Maharastra clothing.

Chapter 6

The Taj Hotel is on Bombay Harbor, opposite the Gateway to India, an ornate monument built to honor the visit of King George V and Queen Mary for the Darbar at Delhi in 1911. In contrast with the dust and disorder in the streets, the lobby of the hotel was immaculate both in architecture and housekeeping. The reception area was full of visitors from the Middle East, who had come to Bombay for medical treatment. Numerous Arab children played relentlessly in the foyer.

Our room was on the seventeenth floor, in a new wing facing the harbor and the Gateway to India. Our balcony overlooked a small park, no more than a quarter of an acre in size. It was difficult to see the green grass, as every inch of both park and side street was covered with hucksters selling their wares. We spent the next hour on the balcony looking down at the comings and goings in the park. There was a continuous throng of humanity, of all sizes, shapes and colors. We were fascinated, but hesitant to go down and observe at closer range.

Later in the afternoon we decided to take a guided tour of the city. Eva was able to secure the services of an employee of the tourist department to escort us around to the sights of Bombay. Our first stop was the Gateway to India. As we stood in front of the gates, it was easy to imagine the pomp and ceremony of welcoming King George V and Queen Mary in Bombay in 1911.

Our guide gave us a brief outline of Indian courtesies. The first was the gesture of folding one's hands, as in prayer, and holding them against the chest and at the same time bowing your head, and saying, "Numa stay," an all-encompassing greeting meaning "Hello," "Thank you," "God bless," etc.

The next item in our introductory course on Indian life was a short lesson on the caste system, which though it is now prohibited by law, is still a very real social fact in many sections of India. For an Indian, everything is related to the caste into which he or she was born. The ideal way of life is sometimes referred to as the "duties of one's class and station (*varna srama dharma*)."

The term "class" (*varna*) is one of the words connoting the caste system peculiar to India. The ancient texts describe four great classes or castes: the *brahmins*, or priests; *the ksatriyas*, warriors and rulers; *the vaisyas*, merchants and farmers; and *the sundras*, peasants and laborers. A fifth class, *panchamas* or "untouchables," includes those whose occupations require them to handle unclean objects. It is believed that the untouchables were assigned to this class because of their non-Aryan origins. This brief outline of the system hardly does justice to the complexity of the modern caste system. The classical works on *dharma* (morality or right conduct) specify the distinct role each is expected to play in the ideal society.

The classical works also outline four ideal stages (*ashrama*), or stations of life, each with its own duties. The first of these is studentship (*brahmacharya*) from initiation at five to eight years of age until marriage; the second, householdership (*grihastha*), when one marries, raises a family, and takes part in society; the third, forest dwelling (*vanaprasta*), after one's children have grown; and the fourth, renunciation (*sanyasa*), when one gives up attachment to all worldly things and seeks spiritual liberation.

These ideal classes and stations apply to males only. The position of women in Hinduism has always been ambiguous: on the one hand, they are venerated as a symbol of the divine, and on the other, they are treated as inferior beings. Women are traditionally expected to serve their husbands and to have no independent interests.

The doctrine of rebirth is a widespread feature of classical Hinduism.

It is the belief in transmigration of souls, or *samsara*, the passage of a soul from body to body as determined by the force of one's actions, or *karma*. In its strictest interpretation, *karma* theory teaches that one's birth into a higher or lower life form or caste, the length of one's life, and the quality of one's experiences are determined by the actions of one's previous existences. This is modified in popular understanding, but it has been a strong influence on most Hindus throughout history. The goal of every devout Hindu is liberation, release from the cycle of death and rebirth. It is typically to be achieved by working out those karmic residues which have already begun to mature, as well as following certain practices to ensure that no further residues are produced to cause future rebirths. The practices by which one may achieve this are frequently termed yoga, and the theory of liberation is the core of Indian philosophy.

The Hindu deities are at first very confusing and their significance is hard to understand. The two great theistic movements within Hinduism are Vaishnavism, the cult of Vishnu, and Shaivism, or the cult of Shiva. Hindu belief, however, usually holds that the universe is populated by a multitude of gods. To some extent these gods share the features of the godhead, but in other ways they behave much as humans do, and are related to each other as humans are. In this respect they are like the gods of the ancient Greeks. For example, the supreme gods, Brahma, Vishnu, Shiva, and others, are often viewed as acting through their relationships with female deities. These female consorts to the deities are called *shakti*. Other well-known gods are said to be relatives of a supreme god; Ganesha, for example, the elephant-headed god, is a son of Shiva and Parvati. Kali, or Durga, the consort of Shiva, is worshipped widely throughout India in the autumn. Hanuman, the monkey-faced god, is depicted in many shrines, and, along with Lakshmi, Vishnu's wife, is among the most important deities associated with Vaishnavism. The sets of gods recognized by different sects are by no means exclusively their own; they may be just as important to other sects.

The forms of worship comprise home worship, temple worship, and a kind of congregational worship very like that practiced in Christian churches in the West. However, this form is rare in India.

Home worship typically involves purification of the living area through fire, water, and the drawing of symbolic diagrams. Depending on class and status, Hindus perform the rites in different ways, are assigned different roles in them, and may perform them more or less often. The rites involve offering food, flowers, or incense to the deity, together with the recitation of appropriate sacred words or texts. An especially important ritual is known as *sraddha*, in which Indian males symbolically support their dead fathers, grandfathers, and great-grandfathers in other worlds, by offering water and balls of rice; this ritual dates from Vedic times. The worshipper requires the services of a priest on this occasion, as for other life-cycle ceremonies such as birth, initiation, marriage, and death.

In temple worship the priests are in charge, although the devotee may participate in the reading of certain hymns or prayers and may give flowers or money directly to the god. The image of the god is believed to be the god, and the cycle of worship in a temple centers on the daily life of the god, involving preparation of the god for worship—waking him with bells, purifying him with incense, bathing, dressing, and feeding him. The worshipper comes to the temple to view the god (*darshana*) and to receive the food (*prasada*) that the god has touched. As in the cycle of an ordinary person, special days occur in the cycle of the god of the temple, and on these days special ceremonies are held. These are frequently the times of festivals and may involve elaborate ceremonies: pilgrimages of vast numbers of devotees, processions bearing the god's image through the city or countryside, and special music, plays, and dances for the occasion.

There are seven sacred cities of Hinduism: Varnasi (Benares), Hardwar, Ayodhya, Dwarka, Mathura, Kanchipuram, and Ujjain. Other important places of pilgrimage include Madurai, Gaya, Prayaga, Tirputati, and Puri. Each of these places has one or more temples where annual festivals are celebrated, attracting large numbers of pilgrims.

Certain festival days are celebrated throughout India on a day fixed according to the Hindu lunisolar calendar. The most prominent of these festivals is Divali, the "Festival of Lights," which occurs in October or November, when lamps are placed around the house to welcome Lakshmi, the goddess of prosperity. Holi, a spring festival, is held in February or March, and is a day of riotous fun-making; this frequently involves temporary suspension of caste and social distinctions, and practical jokes are the order of the day. In the fall a ten-day period is set aside to honor the Mother Goddess, culminating in Dashara, the tenth day, a day of processions and celebrations. This festival is extremely important in Bengal, where it is known as "Durga Puja."

After our brief introduction to Indian customs, castes, and religions we remained somewhat puzzled and confused. However, we were now very aware that Indian society was complex and vastly different from our own.

As our guide drove away from the gates, she pointed out another Indian custom; a mark on the forehead, which distinguished a married woman. She added that the mark was now often used as a cosmetic marking, and did not necessarily distinguish a married woman from an unmarried one, but that if the lady had a red streak in the center of the parting of her hair, she was definitely married.

The masses of people on the streets, the animals, cars, trucks, three-wheelers, two-wheelers, men walking hand in hand with each other, women sitting sidesaddle on the rear of a motorized two-wheeler—cows lying down at a main intersections, the environment filled with a multitude of smells and noisy car horns, blaring bus and truck horns—all of this kept us busy as we attempted to listen to our guide while at the same time looking around in wonder, not wanting to miss a moment of the drama outside the small car.

At each and every traffic stop, our guide had to interrupt her commentary to concentrate on driving in the unbelievably chaotic traffic. She told us that more than five hundred dialects are spoken in Bombay, and fifty different newspapers are printed daily in the city. She mentioned the Parsi religion. There are over 170,000 Parsis, more than 100,000 of whom live in Bombay. They are descendants of Persian Zoroastrians who fled their native land in the tenth century, to escape the persecution of the Muslim majority, and they have preserved, almost unchanged, the beliefs and customs of their ancestors. They respect the ancient prohibitions against the contamination of the sacred elements of fire, water, and earth; their lives are governed by rituals and sacrifice that deal with every aspect of life from birth to death; and they practice the stringent code of morality laid down by Zoroaster. Death is regarded as the ultimate impurity, and Parsis refuse to defile the earth with burial; instead, the body is exposed within a circular, unroofed tower, called a *dakhma*, where it is devoured by vultures.

The Parsis are a closed community and permit neither intermarriage nor proselytization by other faiths. They are noted for their wealth and generosity; they have founded many hospitals, orphanages and schools. On our future trips to South India we became very knowledgeable of the Parsis' philanthropy.

Our next stop was a Jain temple. It was tucked in behind other buildings, off the street, and without a guide we would never have known it was there. The Jains are a small religious group, comprising no more than one or two percent of the population of India. They dress entirely in white, and are very strict in their vegetarian dietary laws: they do not, for example, eat root vegetables as they contain tiny organisms. Likewise, they wear masks so as not to breathe in tiny organisms which they fear will kill them.

On entering the small temple we were dazzled by the brightness of a jeweled necklace around the neck of one of the statues of the gods. We were only allowed into the entranceway, and as is customary in all temples in India, we had to remove our shoes before entering the temple from the street.

Next we visited the house where Mahatma Gandhi resided for a few years when he returned to India from South Africa in the early 1920s. His residence is now a museum of his early life. On entering the house

I was mesmerized by a framed inscription, in English, of the "Seven Social Sins" which Gandhi wrote in 1924. These sins would be seen, by me, in every government office I visited over the next few years. The seven social sins were:

1. Politics without principle
2. Wealth without work
3. Commerce without morality
4. Education without character
5. Pleasure without conscience
6. Science without humanity
7. Worship without sacrifice

The house was austerely furnished; comforts were minimal, and luxuries nonexistent, just as I would have envisioned. There was an excellent historical diorama depicting the Mahatma's life.

The Hanging Gardens were close by, and we decided to visit this famous botanical display. I was not impressed with the maintenance and order of the facility, and the unruly crowds of people caused both Eva and me some concern. On our return to the hotel we decided to rest and attempt to absorb what we had seen.

We soon discovered that, even though we were exhausted from the heat, jet lag, and the overwhelming effect of so many surprising new impressions, we were still unable to relax. We sat on our balcony, looking down into the park, and after a while, we decided to go down and explore.

As we left the hotel grounds, we were instantly surrounded by multitudes of hucksters, young and old, pressing in on us from all sides, proffering their wares and insisting, "It is very good, sir! I will give you the best price!" At first I tried to discourage them by repeatedly stating that I was not interested in what they were selling. But that strategy was to no avail; I soon learned that if you walked on without looking, completely ignoring them, they would leave you alone. We walked towards

Bombay, September 1979

the Gates of India, thinking we would take a look at the harbor. Sitting in front of one of the pillars was a dirty, decrepit old man, with a small wicker basket and a flute lying by his callused bare feet. He immediately addressed us.

"Please, sir, do you want to see my cobra? He is a very smart cobra."

"No," I replied.

"Well, sir," he continued, "you will be surprised at what he does."

I walked on, but Eva was intrigued, and wanted to see what the cobra could do, and even take a picture. I told the old man that I would have to go and get my camera. "No problem, sir," he assured me. "Please do."

I hurried back to our room for the camera. When I returned to the park Eva was standing in front of the snake charmer, and as I approached he beckoned me to come stand beside him. Soon we were surrounded by Indians, at least a hundred, but it seemed more like a thousand. We could hardly breathe, let alone move. The old man lifted the lid off the basket, picked up his flute and started to play. At once, the cobra emerged, raising its head at least two feet above the basket. Both of us were frightened. I didn't dare move. I activated my camera and took numerous continuous pictures.

The old man then introduced me to his mongoose, which was tied to one of his baskets; next he picked up a gunny sack, untied it, and held it out to me, saying, "Please sir, fetch a small snake from the bag and throw it to my mongoose."

"No, thank you," I replied, but before I knew it, the old man had turned his mongoose loose and was throwing small snakes at our feet. Eva and I jumped back and she uttered a frightened scream. At this the crowd roared with laughter.

"What do I owe you?" I asked, hoping to pay him and escape.

"Well, sir," he replied, "these small snakes are very expensive, and I have demonstrated longer than usual. Five hundred rupees would be in order."

"Pay him," Eva said, when she saw me hesitate. I told her the man was asking for too much. (The exchange rate was three rupees to the

Diary of a Miracle

Canadian dollar at the time.) By now the crowd had started closing in on us, and I became frightened. All I could see were brown faces; ours were the only white faces in the park. How could I refuse to pay? I opened my wallet and, giving him 300 rupees, I grabbed Eva's hand and we started to make our way back to the hotel through the crush of people. The more we tried to push our way out of the crowd, the more they tried to hold us back.

The old man was still calling after us, in a loud voice that everyone could hear, "Please, sir, you have not given enough, you still owe me more rupees." Finally we reached the perimeter of the crowd, and hurried toward to the hotel. The doorman had witnessed some of these events, and as we entered the building he asked us what had happened. When I told him that I had refused to pay 500 rupees, a broad smile appeared on his face; even his moustache appeared to be laughing. "Sir," he said, " you paid him too much. The usual fee is two or three rupees. He will be able to retire for a month." With that we started to laugh at ourselves, too. The old man was indeed a smart businessman.

Chapter 7

We woke early Friday morning, expecting to depart for Madras. Eva walked out onto the balcony and hurriedly called to me, laughing, "Look, they are doing their laundry. You can't see the green grass…" She paused, then suddenly exclaimed, "You won't believe what I'm seeing. The grass is moving, no, the white washing is actually people. They must have slept there all night." By now I had joined her on the balcony and together we stood in awe, watching the grass slowly becoming green again as the people awakened and stood up, the women adjusting their white saris and the men their *dhotis* (a white loincloth worn by Hindu men).

"I am sorry, sir," the Indian Airlines agent reported to us when I stopped by her desk in the lobby of the hotel. "Indian airlines went on strike last evening. We don't know when the flights will be resumed. Please check with me tomorrow morning." I returned to tell Eva that we would be spending at least one more day in Bombay.

I then experienced the Indian telephone system. It was almost impossible, I discovered, to make a simple phone call to Madras to let our Rotarian colleague, Krish Chitale, know that our flight was delayed and we would not be arriving as planned. After several futile minutes on the phone I decided that discretion was the better part of valor, and laid the receiver down.

We spent the day relaxing by the pool, and walking the side streets browsing the merchants' stalls, which were filled with wood carvings, clothes of every description, snake purses made from cobra skins, bells, trinkets, figures of gods and goddesses, and a multitude of other odds and ends.

On Saturday, when I enquired at the Indian Airlines desk again, I was told that we should make plans to be at the airport by noon. There would be a flight to Madras, but the agent didn't know the exact departure time. I asked when she thought we should leave the hotel. Her response was brisk and to the point. "Immediately, " she said. "Now, sir, would be the time." We packed without delay, and checked out of the hotel at 10:30 a.m.

The taxi ride to the airport was enjoyable, but it was extremely hot and humid. The driver was talkative and gave us his expanded reflections on Bombay, telling us some of the same stories and anecdotes as our tourist guide. We arrived at the domestic terminal, which, unlike the international terminal at which we had arrived seventy-two hours previously, was in a state of disrepair. Once again we were swarmed by baggage carriers when we stepped out of the taxi. It was raining. Two baggage handlers took command of our luggage without my consent, and we were ushered into the waiting area like puppets on a string.

We wish to check in, please," I told the attendant.

"I'm sorry, no check-in at this time. Please sit here. You will be informed when it is proper for you to check in your baggage." With that he held out his hand and demanded ten rupees. I put six rupees into his dirty palm.

"That's all, sir," I said. "One rupee per bag," I read out to him, pointing to the sign over the door, which clearly stated the charges.

The bench we occupied was dirty and stained, and looked old enough to have been manufactured for Queen Victoria's visit. As I looked around, all I could see were Indians sleeping on the floor, children sitting talking endlessly, and infants having their daily bowel ritual on the dirty marble floor. Mothers had made small dung fires and were busy cooking. Sprinkled here and there were Middle Eastern people in brightly colored headgear, the men in flowing white robes and the women gowned in bright colors, and Muslim ladies in their long black dresses, their children following every move they made.

Bombay, September 1979

I looked at Eva. We were both asking ourselves the same questions: "What are we doing?" and "Why are we here?" Outside it was now raining intensely. Inside, the humidity was on the rise, and the heat was unendurable. I looked at my watch; it was now noon.

I approached the check-in area, which was vacant. A sign was posted, which read, "There will be a flight to Madras this evening, check-in time is unknown at this time." I was to become very familiar with the sign over the next several hours. Every thirty minutes or so I found myself looking at it, hoping, I guess, that the message would be different, though I knew it was not. In the intervals we sat and stared at all the different sites around our bench. The dung cooking fires did not smell any better, the cooking pots were still active, children were still talking, playing or sleeping. The men were still sleeping on the dirty marble floor, and infants and young children were still attending to their normal bowel functions unimpeded. Between laughing and crying to myself, I continued to wonder what on earth we were doing there. Everything we had experienced in India up to this point now looked, in retrospect, quite wonderful. We were certainly adventuring into the unknown, as we waited for our flight to Madras. As I looked at Eva with her white missionary hat in place, I felt like a real outsider. I wondered what the natives thought of us.

My 5:30 p.m. walk to check-in was finally productive. The sign had been changed. It now read "Check-in will commence at 6:00 p.m. for flight to Madras." I returned quickly and relayed the good news to Eva. We then proceeded with our six pieces of luggage to the check-in area. We were fifth in line, and naively confident that things would now move speedily. We were unaware that we would have to stand there and wait for another hour before the complicated and frustrating procedure of checking our luggage would even begin.

"You are forty kilos over the allowance," the slim, moustached Indian informed me. "Take this slip to the cashier and return to me." I asked where the cashier might be found. "Upstairs," was his brief reply.

I left Eva at the side of the counter while I went to ferret out the cashier. Every person I asked gave me different directions. Finally I found what I thought was a security guard, who turned out to be a military official. He told me to "follow the stairs to the next floor, turn right, then left and at the end of the corridor is the cashier's office."

"That will be 150 rupees, sir," the cashier said.

"Do you take American Express?"

"We are not familiar with the card, and besides that we only take rupees." I scrutinized the contents of my wallet, shocked to find that all I had was one 50-rupee note. I quickly returned to Eva, who was still patiently reading her book at the side of the check-in counter.

"No money," I said, attempting to take a humorous view of the matter. Eva went through her wallet, but she too was out of cash.

"I'll cash some travelers' checks," she said. I attempted to give her directions to the cashier's office on the second floor, and off she went. I looked at my watch; it was 6:50 p.m.

The next time I looked it was 7:20, and Eva was still not back. Where was she? The Indian Airlines agent chose that moment to remind me that the flight would be departing at 8:15 p.m. and that it would take considerable time to pass through security. My frustration was mounting by the minute. Where was Eva? What had happened? At 7:35 p.m., I turned around and there she stood with a broad smile on her face. "You'll never believe what I went through. I couldn't locate the cashier's office. Several people tried to help, but they all gave me different directions. Eventually I found an old man who spoke very good English, and he took me upstairs, direct to the cashier's office. However, when we got there he explained that the cashier isn't permitted to cash any foreign travelers' checks or change any currency, and that I had to go downstairs again, to the money changer."

We paid the agent, and in return we received several pages of paper which certified that our excess baggage was now allowed on board the plane.

Fortunately, we passed through security without encountering any more pointless delays. Shortly before 8:21 p.m., we boarded the DC9

Bombay, September 1979

and were shown to cramped seats at the rear of the plane. I sat wondering what the situation would be in Madras. I had had no contact since the telex I had received in late August asking me to postpone my trip, as the government of India had not made up their minds whether to allow measles vaccine into India.

As we landed in Madras it became evident that the humidity was high. Outside the plane, the windows were draped in misty curtains. We waited till the plane was nearly empty. "What do we do now?" Eva asked.

I tried to reassure her. "There must be lots of hotels in Madras. We'll make out okay. Don't worry." Descending from the plane, I was wondering where we would sleep that night.

I really didn't envision that history would be made over the next three weeks, but that was how it turned out. I was just a small part of Rotary's India story, which had been initiated by District Governor Bud Crookes of District 707 and Governor P.J. from District 320, Coimbatore. I was to be the unknown catalyst, setting in motion events that would make medical history in the subcontinent of India.

Chapter 8

Two other planes had arrived just before ours, one from New Delhi and the other from Calcutta. The baggage area was old and dirty, crowded and confused. There was only one carousel for the three flights that had arrived almost simultaneously, and all of the passengers, about 300 people, were trying to get into an area that had the capacity for 200, maximum. Eva was talking with the only other white woman, the wife of a Lutheran missionary.

It was impossible to reach the rickety baggage carousel because of the congestion. The numbers present made the temperature unbearable. A thermometer registered 100 degrees Fahrenheit, and coupled with the humidity it felt like 110 degrees Fahrenheit. I joined Eva and the missionary's wife in conversation. She told us that she had been in South India for fifteen years, and she assured us that we would enjoy the experience. Suddenly, there was a tap on my shoulder. I turned, and was greeted by a short, moderately stout Indian.

"I am president C.T. of the Madras club," he said. "Welcome to Madras." With these words he garlanded Eva and me with flowers. Indicating another smiling man in the group who stood just behind him, he added, "This is your host, Krish Chitale."

Before I could say hello, Mr. Chitale asked, in a loud voice that everybody close by could hear, "And how many wives do you have?"

"Only one," I replied. And with that, Chitale asked for our baggage stubs and sent another Rotarian in the group to fetch our luggage.

The drive from the airport to Krish's house was filled with talk about

· Madras, September 1979 ·

the measles project. As we climbed out of the car, Krish said that we would continue the conversation tomorrow.

The entrance to his home was magnificent. It was like a picture from *Better Homes and Gardens*. Servants took our bags and showed us to our room, which was off the main sitting area on the main floor. After we cleaned up, we entered the sitting room. Krish and C.T. were deep in conversation.

Krish was an impressive-looking Indian man, about five foot eight, with curly hair just starting to grey. His demeanor was quiet; he seemed both sincere and fair-minded. He was direct in conversation, always stating his point of view quickly and concisely. He never hesitated to express his views, even if there was a chance that they might offend the listener. C.T., on the other hand, was short, no more than five foot five, moderately rotund, with a happy sense of humor and a constantly smiling, rounded face. His hair was sparse and seemed to be quickly disappearing.

As we sat down, Krish turned to me and without preamble asked, "Who paid your way?"

Taken aback, I quickly replied, "We paid our own way—if it makes any difference."

"It certainly does," replied Krish. "It means that you mean business." With that, he extended his hand in friendship.

I soon guided the conversation to the subject of measles.

"That will be handled tomorrow," Krish replied. "What will you have to drink? A brandy, perhaps?" I could hardly believe my ears. It was my understanding that all Indians were teetotalers.

"Nothing," was my answer. "Perhaps Eva would like a cup of tea."

"That will be fine," Krish said, and gave the order to the servant. He approached a cabinet, and opening the bottom drawer he took out a fine bottle of brandy and placed it on the top. He then set about pouring two brandies, one for himself and one for President C.T.

"Perhaps," I said thoughtfully, "I will have a brandy."

Krish looked me straight in the eye and in a terse voice replied, "Ken, let's get one thing clear. I won't try to impress you and you won't try to impress me. I only offer what I have. If you want it, fine, if you don't, fine. Let's not try and impress each other." With those words, we understood each other, and established the basis for a friendship that still exists.

The brandy was excellent and the conversation stimulating. At bedtime, Krish told us that breakfast would be at 8:30 a.m., and wished us a good night.

I was awakened by a discreet knock on our bedroom door.

"Morning coffee, sir. I have it with me."

I looked at my watch. It was 6:30 a.m. A figure entered the darkened bedroom, set a tray down on a table, and left as quickly and quietly as he came. I fell asleep again immediately.

The next thing I heard was the sound of Eva entering the bedroom. Waking me from a deep comfortable sleep, she exclaimed, "You won't believe it! They eat with their hands, except for the eggs."

"What do you mean?"

"I've just come from having a wonderful breakfast. They eat with their hands, and don't use a fork or a knife." Eva gave me a rundown of the breakfast menu while I was shaving, and it all sounded so delicious that I rushed even faster.

On entering the dining room on the next level, I was greeted with "Good morning, uncle!" coming from a most attractive sixteen-year-old girl, whose name, I later learned, was Chinku. It was the endearing Indian custom for children and teenagers to address friends of the family, or visitors to their home, as "uncle" and "auntie." "Daddy will be here shortly, uncle. Please sit down!"

My place at the table was obvious: there was only one place set with a knife and fork. This was the first and last time that a knife and fork were placed before me in the Chitales' home. Being called uncle made me feel very much at home, and I decided that in future I would eat at Indian tables in the correct Indian manner.

Krish appeared at the table, and breakfast began. We ate *puri*, which are like a puffy light doughnut, made from hand-ground flour, and fried in oil; *dosa*, which resembles pancakes, except that they are very thin, almost like French crepes, and are eaten with vegetables or chutney; and *idlis*, slightly sour, steamed rice cakes, also eaten with a fresh vegetable sauce, called *sambar*. With all of this, one drinks coffee—in the Chitale household, instant coffee was served. This was the first of many breakfasts that Eva and I would share with the Chitales over the next twenty-one years.

"Now, let's get down to work, Ken," said Krish. "There is so much we have to talk about and do over the next few days."

This was the true beginning of the work I had come to India to do: our objective was the immunization of 68,000 Indian children with measles antigen.

Krish went on, "The state government is very slow to accept even the concept of measles, and the federal government in Delhi is the same. There are a lot of formidable problems you and I must face, and solve, if we are to be successful, so please have patience. Hopefully, we will overcome." Krish then handed me an outline of our schedule for the next few days. I was soon to discover that Indians are very formal and hesitant until you really get to know them and they develop a trust in you. I found that it took Krish almost forty-eight hours to be able to speak to me forthrightly and frankly. After that, our friendship grew quickly.

Chapter 9

After breakfast, Krish filled me in on the status of the project. All was not well. The state ministry of health was reluctant to endorse the project, in part because the federal ministry of health in Delhi was still fighting the war of the Edmonston versus the Swartz strain of vaccine, even though Dr. Henderson of the World Health Organization in Geneva had advised New Delhi health officials by telex to accept the project. Dr. Henderson had forwarded a copy of his telex to Bill Nurse in Whitby on September 7. Bill, in turn, sent on a copy of the telex to Madras for my information.

Dr. Henderson's telex stated: "The Edmonston strain is a further attenuated strain having reactogenicity similar to the Swartz strain, and is widely used in the tropics with good effect." He further stated that he had telexed World Health in New Delhi advising the government to accept the project.

A follow-up telex by Dr. Henderson on September 11 stated:

> We are informed that the Drug Collector, Government of India, has not as yet approved the Edmonston further attenuated strain of measles. An urgent opinion is being sought in response to your request, but this is an internal government process and approval of this vaccine by World Health does not oblige government to accept it. We continue to hope that this will be resolved satisfactorily.

Madras, September 1979

Krish then handed me the telex that Bill Nurse had sent me on September 14, which stated: "Health Ministry approved the shipment planned for 20 September." Krish said that, unfortunately, only the day after receiving the telex, the ministry had changed their minds. He went on to say that the local doctors, including Rotarian doctors, were opposed to the project because they stood to lose their medical fee in dispensing the vaccine.

I looked at Krish and exclaimed, "I can't believe what I am hearing."

"The truth is, Ken—welcome to India." There was a pause and then he continued, "If you believe in this as much as I do, then we shall overcome all adversities."

I had a great deal of difficulty in accepting the idea that some Rotarian doctors were against the proposed measles project for financial considerations of their own. India was indeed a puzzle that would become more perplexing and difficult as time passed. I was truly a North American, believing that every country in the world must support certain widely accepted humanitarian ideals, such as helping the poor and destitute. Fairness to all is important too, of course, including both the privileged and the others, but surely the most important principle is compassion for the underprivileged and the poor.

I asked Krish about storage of the vaccine. I was concerned about this issue as the vaccine is very heat sensitive and has to be stored below 8 degrees Celsius in order to maintain its potency. I wondered about that in a country with such a warm climate. Krish's answer was simple, to the point, and not reassuring.

"That's another problem. The electricity goes off every morning at 7:45 a.m. and remains off for one to three hours a time. However, we will look into storage facilities tomorrow. Today is a day of relaxation and I have a few things lined up for you. C.T. will join us later on; however, first I want to introduce you to the pediatric institute, a government hospital."

"Wonderful. I look forward to seeing a pediatric institution." Little did I realize that it would be an experience that would disturb me for the rest of my life.

Krish drove his car, a large, vintage, North American-looking type called an "Ambassador." The vehicle was made in India; it was heavy and lacked any form of springs or shock absorbers. The driving time was less than twenty-five minutes. On the way our conversation returned constantly to the measles project, despite the difficulty of talking over the incessant noise of traffic. The streets were very crowded and busy, with continual sounding of horns, and motorists driving in an erratic manner. I mentioned the traffic problems to Krish.

He laughed and said, "This is a holiday, Ken. This traffic is very sparse. Just wait until tomorrow (Monday). You'll see the typical Madras driving, which is undisciplined and rude."

The Institute of Pediatrics was an old building, built at the turn of the century. As we entered the hospital, I couldn't help noticing the extreme lack of maintenance, combined with poor housekeeping. Unfortunately, I was constantly making comparisons with our hospitals in Canada. I realized this was a wrong attitude to take, but I am only human and this was my first morning in Madras. It is easier now, in hindsight, to comprehend the problems the medical staff had to contend with, but my dismay at that moment only shows how completely overwhelmed I was by India, South India in particular. The chief of pediatrics met us at the door. His name I do not remember. South Indians have particularly long names, and lack a surname. This, coupled with their peculiar inflection and cadence, makes it very difficult to grasp what they are saying. It takes a matter of days to tune in to the local speech patterns enough to be able to completely understand what they are saying.

As he spoke, it gradually became apparent to me that he was talking about the pathology of meningitis as diagnosed in South India. I understood that we were going to visit an intensive care unit for convulsing children. As we walked towards the unit, I once again noticed the lack of adequate housekeeping. Dirt and debris were everywhere. We stopped in front of a ward door marked "Authorized Personnel Only," and entered.

The room was darkened. A small window air-conditioner hummed in

· Madras, September 1979 ·

a window at the far end of the room. The room was approximately twenty by thirty feet in size. Some sixteen cribs were squeezed in side by side, with just enough room for a nurse or doctor to be able to pass between them. The constant moaning and crying of mothers lying on the floor, either beside or under their child's crib, was very disturbing. The chief went on to point out the condition of the various children in the ward: this child was convulsing with tubercular meningitis, that one was convulsing because of tetanus and was in the last stages before dying; another had an unexplained etiology for his meningitis. Here was a child with tubercular meningitis, a child with syphilis, another with meningococcal meningitis. It became apparent that deaths were occurring as we spoke. The odor and the terrible despair in the atmosphere were on the verge of making me feel intensely ill. I looked at Krish. He too looked as if he was contemplating escape from the room. The doctor, seeing our faces, recognized that we had seen enough and ushered us out of the intensive care room.

Our drive back home was extremely quiet. Back at the house, I entered our bedroom and Eva looked at me curiously, then with alarm. "What's the matter? You look terrible—are you ill?"

"Please, Eva, just let me be quiet for a few minutes. I'll be all right."

In a few moments I had regained my composure, and was able to tell her about my visit to the children's ward. I tried to convey to her the impact it had had on me, but it was difficult to talk about. I described the children and how three of them had died while we were present. Their cribs were filled again, almost immediately, by other critically ill children. "I have never experienced such an episode in all of my twenty-five years in medicine," I told her. "I will never forget this horrendous experience."

We sat for a few minutes and then joined the family in the living room. In the open area above us, I could hear a tinkling of bells, interspersed with a low chant that continued for some time.

"That is my wife, Susheila, doing her morning prayers in the *pujai* room. She will be finished in a few minutes and then she will join us," said Krish. It was explained to us that the *pujai* room is a special place in Indian homes, where religious images are kept, and prayers said.

A moment later a warm, lovable-looking woman in her early fifties entered the room, dressed in a beautiful sari. She had an obvious limp. Smiling broadly, she said to Eva and me, "Welcome to Madras. I am sorry that I didn't stay up to meet you last evening. However, you did arrive very late. Please, accept my apologies."

"Of course," we assured her. Susheila sat down beside Eva and they quickly became absorbed in conversation about their families and children. Susheila became a friend immediately. Her unpretentious nature made both of us feel entirely at home and relaxed.

C.T. arrived and announced that he was going to take us to the opening cricket match between India and Australia, and so, after getting organized for the outing, we set off.

The cricket match was indeed an experience. There were over 100,000 people in the stadium, which had been built and given to the city of Madras by C.T.'s father-in-law. I must confess that the rules of the match were given to me by six or seven different Rotarians, and between attempting to understand their accents and understanding the rules of the game, I was out to lunch.

However, I did my best to appear to have understood the rules of the game. It was very, very hot: 40 degrees Celsius, with 90 percent humidity.

At the first tea break C.T. and Krish escorted me to the upper deck of the stadium and into the private enclosed box of C.T.'s father-in-law. To my amazement I was offered a gin and tonic and introduced to C.T.'s father-in-law, along with the chief of police and other important dignitaries, including the High Commissioners of Australia and England. For a few moments I was speechless. Earlier, Krish had told me that the only criminal offense that was non-bailable was liquor possession. The state of Tamil Nadu had a very strict and strictly enforced prohibition law. Liquor consumption or possession was illegal everywhere in the state of Tamil Nadu.

Madras, September 1979

Three days later, accompanied by Krish, Eva and I went to a state government office to apply for a temporary liquor permit. We swore an affidavit that we were addicted to alcohol, and in return we were given a four-week permit, which was stamped in our passports. This allowed each of us to buy six bottles of alcoholic spirits from a government wine merchant.

The purchasing of our bottles of Indian gin and Scotch whiskey was another unique experience. One night after our evening meal, Krish drove us to the wine merchant's. He parked his car some two blocks away and gave us our instructions of what to buy. Eva and I quickly walked the darkened two blocks and entered an empty establishment. There was a long counter behind which were several groups of Indians. As we entered, the official boss beckoned us to approach the first group of two. "What is your preference?" he asked, in a very heavy, almost incomprehensibly accented voice.

"Two whiskey, two gin," I replied.

"I am sorry, sir, please speak a little slower and plainer, as I have great difficulty in understanding your request."

I smiled at him, patiently. Little did he realize the difficulty I was having in understanding him.

"Two McDowell whiskey," I pronounced very slowly, "and two gin."

"Thank you, sir, that is entirely understandable."

He then waved me on to the next group of two behind the counter. I saw as I turned that he had written our order on a piece of old paper and had passed it on to the next wicket. The two behind the wicket read our order intently and after a few moments one of them asked, "Do you have a permit, sir?"

"Yes," I replied, and handed him our passports.

He cautiously perused our passports for several minutes, before announcing, "All is in order, sir," and waving us on to the next group of two behind the counter in yet another wicket.

"That will be 45 rupees, sir," he said as he pushed a massive sheet of paper towards us, with a pen. I assumed we must sign, and as I picked up the pen he authoritatively exclaimed, "No, sir, not now, only when we have delivered the goods." Hurriedly he took our money and passed it on to his assistant; his duty, apparently, was to count the money, write a note as to how much change we were to receive, and return the amount to his colleague. Calculators were unheard of in this establishment. Longhand calculations had to be made, checked, and rechecked before the slip of paper was handed to the next wicket.

As I gazed ahead, I could happily see that we had almost reached the end of our elaborate transaction. It had only taken twenty minutes to get this far. Eva quietly whispered, "Patience, patience."

Finally, we received our change and moved to the last wicket. Here two clerks examined each bottle before wrapping our purchases in old newspaper; then at last they handed them over. As we left the empty store, I quietly said to Eva, "Thank God we were the only ones in the store."

As we approached the darkened car, Krish quickly started it, and we drove off, without headlights until we reached the main road. "One must always be cautious," he said, anxiously. "As I told you, an alcohol offense in this state is the only offense that is non-bailable." As we entered a small street, Krish once again darkened his headlights and drove into a darkened driveway.

"Two whiskey," he said, and Eva passed two bottles from the back seat. Krish was only gone for a short period, and once again we were on our way without lights.

This would be repeated four more times before we returned home. Later on, as we sat and had a whiskey (imported Scotch), Krish once again stressed the importance of taking extreme caution when delivering whiskey. I am sure the bootleggers in North America during Prohibition took far fewer precautions than we did that September night in Madras.

Chapter 10

Monday morning, September 17, arrived. As usual, the electricity was off from 7:46 a.m. till 9:16 a.m. The knowledge that the measles vaccine was very heat sensitive, coupled with fact that there continued to be constant blackouts of hydro power, which sometimes went on for days, was causing my anxiety level to rise. The vaccine would be arriving within ten days, and there were still too many unanswered questions. Krish seemed philosophical. There were more pressing problems, he said, that had to be solved first. The storage problem could be dealt with later.

He listed the main difficulties:

1) Would the Indian Ministry of Health give their permission for the vaccine to enter India?
2) Would the Tamil Nadu government allow the vaccine to arrive and be stored in Madras?
3) Would the medical doctors of the area, both Rotarian and non-Rotarian, endorse the program and lend their support?
4) Was the Rotary Club of Madras significantly behind the project?
5) Would we be able to get our message across to the five million people of Madras and the forty-five million of the state of Tamil Nadu?

The more I pondered these questions, the more confused I became. The questions I had asked myself in the beginning came back and nagged at me again: "What am I doing in Madras? Why me? Why not some else? Is this project an impossible dream?" That morning I committed myself to the project once again. Without any guarantee of success, I knew I had to travel down the long and frustrating road of attempting to introduce measles vaccine into India, a country that neither knew nor cared about the seriousness of the communicable disease called measles.

I felt certain that Krish and the collection of Rotarians around him were sincere, dedicated, and committed to this project of immunizing the children and infants of South India against the dread scourge of red measles. I soon felt very comfortable with them. C.T., whom I had met on my arrival to Madras; Kumar, a young Rotarian involved in the chemical business; Gopal who worked for Air France (and so I called him Gopal Air France); K.V. Shetty, an executive of a piston manufacturer; Dr. C.R.R. Pilay, a past district governor of Rotary District 320—these were the initial core group. As we worked for the acceptance of the project, numerous other Rotarians became involved.

Government approval was the priority issue. Krish and I had a series of meetings with numerous government health officials on an almost daily basis. The first was merely an exploratory meeting. Accordingly, they were very polite and very noncommittal.

The director of health services for the government of Tamil Nadu was cool, aloof and uninterested in what we had to say. He sat behind his desk and appeared to be distant. I got to know him very well as we visited him on at least three occasions over a ten-day period. Behind his desk was what I called his "scoreboard." On this board in chalk were listed the number of deaths for the previous four-week period from such illnesses as cholera, typhoid, malaria, gastrointestinal tract disorders, polio, and whooping cough. Deaths from measles and its complications were not listed. On my third visit to his office I remarked on that fact and asked him the reason. His answer was sharp, crisp and to the point, at least in his mind. "Dr. Hobbs, you see, measles is not a reportable disease and is not part of the federal government's expanded program for immunization." Enough said, my concerns were answered!

Madras, September 1979

There are four medical schools in Madras. I had the privilege of visiting two of them. They were associated with very large government hospitals. The hospitals are so huge that it is difficult to assess the number of inpatients at any one time. The main medical school has a 10,000-bed hospital associated with the school. As we toured the hospital facility with the dean, I was impressed with their cardiac care unit. However, many areas of the hospital lacked adequate housekeeping. Stray cats walked up and down the corridors, birds were ever-present in some of the wards, as window screens were conspicuous by their absence. At the end of our tour the dean asked if I had any special interest. I mentioned that I would love to see a case of betel nut carcinoma. This is a carcinoma that appears in people who are addicted to chewing betel nut (the nut grows on a type of palm tree; it is ground and other components, usually tobacco, are added, and the mixture is placed in the user's mouth between the cheek and lower teeth. Prolonged exposure to this irritant produces a very serious form of carcinoma).

"That it is not impossible," the dean replied. He picked up a phone and called the outpatient department. Within a very short period of time, eighteen cases of "betel nut carcinomas," in various stages, were presented to me. This was indeed a very interesting morning for me. I am perhaps the only graduate of Medicine '55 of the University of Western Ontario who has ever seen not one, but eighteen, such cases.

As we took our leave of the dean I expressed my sincere pleasure in the privilege of my visit to this very large institution.

We drove to another government office, at the Red Fort Building. Here I was introduced into the state government's Secretary in Charge of Medical Education. He was pleasant, friendly, but, like all the others, noncommittal. We talked at great length about the seriousness of red measles, and how the disease could be prevented with a single injection of vaccine. His answers were vague; he kept repeating that the state government could not unilaterally make this commitment, before the federal government in New Delhi had set the guidelines. I felt as if I were charting the first trip to the moon all by myself. As we left his office he wished me well.

Outside, Krish expressed his concern. This was an official whose support we had to obtain, he said. Perhaps by further visits we might win him over to the idea of the project. We then proceeded to Krish Chitale's own office.

His office was on a busy street called Anna Road. Little did I realize that over the next twenty-one years I would be spending a great deal of time at this location. As we approached the small elevator to go to the third floor, the attendant cleared the lift and Krish and I proceeded up by ourselves. The operator of the lift sized me up very thoroughly and meticulously.

As we entered Krish's office we were greeted by his secretary, an older man who wore glasses and tended to squint and feel insecure when he was spoken to by Krish. He sat behind a formal desk, and one could not enter the inner part of the office without first confronting this squinting secretary, who fiercely guarded the lattice push gate that allowed an authorized person to enter. Several years later this quiet insecure secretary gave Krish a great deal of remorse in some personal financial indiscretions.

The sudden activity within the office was amazing. The place was planned on an open concept design, with a private office on your right as you entered and passed the gate. In the open central area ten to twelve technicians bent over drafting tables while a few others were talking with clients or contractors. I was ushered into Krish's private office and boardroom. The secretary presented me with a large file.

"Mr. Chitale wishes you to look at this file, sir, while he is busy. A coffee, sir?"

"No," I replied, "not just now, thank you."

As I perused his file I noticed several telexes he had received recently. Krish had shown me copies of these telexes, but they were important, and as I read them again I contemplated once more whether ours was truly a viable mission. Bill Nurse's message, dated September 14, read:

· Madras, September 1979 ·

> Rec'd telex from Chitale Madras Club stating health minister approved. Shipment planned for 20th September. Bud Crookes awaits your approval. Bill Nurse.

And the telex from Dr. Henderson from WHO, dated 11 September 1979:

> We are informed that the Drug Controller government of India has not yet approved Edmonston further attenuated strain of measles vaccine. An urgent opinion is being sought in response to your requests but this is an internal government process and approval of this vaccine by WHO does not oblige government to accept it. We continue to hope this will be resolved satisfactorily. Henderson, UNISANTE, Geneva.

At the end of the day I went to bed pondering over and over the apparently unsolvable problems we were facing. Would the project go ahead? How could it?

And I kept mulling over what Krish had said to me earlier: "If you believe as much as I do, then we shall overcome all adversities."

Chapter 11

The following day, September 18, I attended the meeting of the Rotary Club of Madras. As I entered the Connemara Hotel, I was thinking of another Canadian Rotarian, James Wheeler Davidson, who had traveled with his wife and daughter, at his own expense, to establish Rotary clubs in Europe, Africa, India and the Far East. Davidson established three main clubs in India in 1928 and 1929: the Rotary clubs of Bombay and Calcutta, and the Rotary Club of Madras in 1929. As I entered I felt indeed very privileged to follow, fifty years later, in the footsteps of such a Rotarian.

The Rotary Club of Madras has more than 175 members. The previous evening Eva and I had attended a meeting of the board of directors, all of whose members had gone out of their way to offer us a friendly hand of welcome; their warmth made us feel that we belonged. The meeting had been in this same room of the hotel, and as I stood with Krish now, I recalled the previous evening. After the meeting, the hotel personnel had stood guard at all entrances to the room while President C.T. opened a bottle of Scotch and offered everyone a drink. Krish had whispered to me that this was the first such welcome ever extended to any Rotarian—C.T. was running the risk of being arrested and sent to jail, simply to show us hospitality!

President C.T. now greeted us with warmth and sincerity. He ushered us to the head table. He had asked me to speak, greeting the members of the club and explaining my reason for coming to Madras, and what the measles vaccine project was expected to accomplish. My address was brief and to the point. I reiterated my concern for governmental approval and asked for the club to stand behind Krish and his committee in his valiant effort to immunize 68,000 children against the dread disease of red measles. As I spoke, I had no inkling that my fifteen-minute address was falling on completely deaf ears.

After the meeting, I was approached by a Rotarian pediatrician, whose face expressed grave concern. "Do you realize," he asked, "that this immunization project will endanger the ability of pediatricians to make a living?" Private patients, he explained to me, paid over 30 rupees per injection. (Thirty rupees was equal to $10 Cdn. in 1979—a price that 98 percent of Indians could not even dream of paying.) Our vaccine, he pointed out, which would be administered free of charge, might pose a serious threat to his livelihood.

I was speechless. After thanking him, I walked away, my thoughts in turmoil. I was beginning to see the depth of misunderstanding and opposition I would have to deal with in my determination to change the medical profession and the government's attitudes towards red measles immunization.

Krish scheduled a press conference in his office for the following day. At 10:30 a.m., just before the press conference, a meeting of Rotarians and government officials was held to stress the importance of the project and to attempt to enlist their support. Present were C.T. (V. Chidambaram), Dr. C. Thirugaana, of the Children's Hospital in Madras, Dr. A.S. Padmanabhan, Professor of Pediatrics at the Tanjore Medical College, Dr. S. Anandavavelu, Pondicherry, President A.M. Sharif of the Velore Club, Dr. Jacob John of the Vellore Rotary Club, Dr. M.S. Sundararajan, of the Christian Medical College in Vellore, Dr. Dileep Mathai, Department of Medicine, CMC, Vellore.

At this meeting, certain priorities were established. Children one to five years of age would be immunized first. It was pointed out that every year this age group of the population would be recovered. Therefore, we should be planning a five-year program for suburban and rural areas of Madras; some other stipulated centers would also be considered for the program. It was decided that further technical aspects would be discussed at a future meeting to be held at the Institute of Child Health. Because of the high incidence of tuberculosis in both the urban and rural areas, it was decided that children would be immunized providing no active disease was detected in a pre-immunization medical examination.

The press conference was attended by representatives of *The Hindu*, *U.N.I.*, *The Mail*, *Indian Express* and *P.T.I.* newspapers. Several Rotarians and other interested parties were present. Krish outlined the reasons for the project, and emphatically stated that the vaccine had been used everywhere in the world, including tropical regions such as the Caribbean and several countries in Africa. He stressed the importance of keeping the vaccine in a cold environment in order to protect its potency. Rotarian V.J. Chacko of Spencer's Department Store, he announced that Spencer's Store had consented to allow the vaccine to be stored in their large walk-in freezer lockers. These walk-in lockers were backed up with an automatic generator power supply. The vaccine had to be stored at a constant temperature of between 0 and 8 degrees Celsius. He hoped that the immunization program would save millions of Indian children from measles, an affliction, he emphasized, that was as debilitating and as deadly as smallpox. The safety of the vaccine had been illustrated by the fact that over 85 million children around the world had already been immunized, with no major complications. This would be the first attempt of its kind in India. A feasibility study of measles vaccine would be conducted in two peripheral pediatric centers; and the Indian Medical Association would be holding a meeting with Dr. Hobbs at the Institute of Child Health in the very near future. He concluded by reminding his listeners that 1979, besides being the International Year of the Child, also coincided with the Golden Jubilee of the Rotary Club of Madras, and that this was surely an appropriate time for the initiation of a project of such importance.

The audience was clearly very interested. After Krish had concluded, there were excited murmurs and some applause. During the question-and-answer period, a short man with a dark goatee stood up and offered these comments: "Your project is fine, Dr. Hobbs. You come to Madras

Madras, September 1979

and complete a 68,000-dose program, and then go home and feel that you have done your job. Do you not realize how insufficient that is? Do you realize the significance of measles immunization in the developing world? Are you aware that ten children die each and every minute of every day, day in day out, year in and year out, and five of the ten, half of all these deaths, are due to measles? Perhaps you do not realize that ten children become handicapped every minute of every day from communicable disease that could be prevented by immunization, and that five of these are due to measles. You toss us the bait and then leave, feeling that you have fulfilled your obligation to the children of South India. What are your plans for future measles immunization in South India?"

With this, he sat down. I paused momentarily to collect my thoughts, but I knew I had to try to respond to the very serious question he had raised. "As you know, I cannot and will not commit my Rotary club or Rotary district. The only person I can commit is myself. And I do so now. I promise you that I will do everything I can to make this program work. On my return to Canada I will raise the necessary funds, even if I have to dance on a street corner, to ensure that down the road every child born in this state will be protected against red measles."

To applause, I sat down. After the room had cleared I asked Krish the identity of the little man with the beard. He replied, "That is Dr. Jacob John. He is a Christian originally from the state of Kerala. Christian names are different from Hindu names, hence his name Jacob John. He is a Rotarian from Vellore, a virologist and epidemiologist at the Christian Medical Center there." This institution, Krish added, was established by an American lady missionary working for the Presbyterian Church at the turn of the century. It had originally been reserved for ladies only, but over the past several years had become co-educational. It is one of the top medical schools and research centers in India.

That evening, at Krish's home, I had a chance to speak to Dr. Jacob John at greater length, and in a more relaxed atmosphere. He thanked me for my answer to his question. He had long been interested in measles prevention, he told me; he outlined his past work in certain controlled areas in the Vellore district. I realized as we talked that Dr. Jacob John's path and mine were likely to cross many times in the next several years. (In fact, that is what happened. He and I were chosen by President Carlos Canseco in 1984 to join his committee to set up a program to eradicate poliomyelitis in the world by 2005, the hundredth anniversary of Rotary International. We also served as consultants to the programs committee of The Rotary Foundation from 1987 to 1990.)

Dr. Jacob John became an invaluable asset in the early stages of the project; his contribution was, in part, his campaign to overcome the reluctance of the Indian medical profession to accept measles immunization—a reluctance that was very alarming to me.

His knowledge of the local customs and superstitions of the village people was another important factor in the success of the project. He explained to me that people in the villages regarded measles as a visit from a goddess. Once a goddess visited a home, she could not be interfered with, or she would get revenge by creating havoc, and bringing bad luck on the family. Dr. Jacob John's solution to this problem was to convince the parents that if we immunized their children, they could welcome the goddess to come and visit their household at any time, without fear of any harm coming to anyone in the house. This simple reassurance would become a major factor in our drive to immunize the children in the villages of the state of Tamil Nadu.

One result of our press conference was evident a few days later, when the Indian Medical Association held a symposium on measles. Despite the fact that it was held on a Saturday afternoon, more than two hundred doctors attended, as well as several prominent medical teachers and leaders of the medical community in Madras and the surrounding area. But even more significant was the fact that important leaders of the Indian Health Ministry for the state of Tamil Nadu came to the symposium. These same individuals who had given me the runaround on several occasions now expressed their encouragement for the success of the project.

The statistics presented at this seminar were very enlightening. I learned first-hand from the medical experts that for every 10,000 chil-

· Madras, September 1979 ·

dren born in South India in 1979, there would be 1,000 cases of severe gastroenteritis occurring before their fifth birthday, and that there would be five to ten deaths. There would be countless cases of polio, which would (strangely) not result in significant numbers dying, and there would be six hundred to eight hundred cases of measles, of which thirty to forty children would die. These numbers seemed remarkably low, which confused me until I realized that the systems of reporting and recording the incidence of communicable diseases was not up to North American standards.

One lecturer reemphasized that measles was the greatest killer of children in their first three years of life, and was the third cause of blindness in the first five years of a child's life. I sat on the podium feeling a certain inner warmth; perhaps, I thought, we were getting our message across.

Even though we had received permission to import the vaccine a couple of days after my arrival, Krish and I kept up a continuous pursuit of a broad range of government health officials daily. Eventually, the federal health ministry asked Krish and me to come to a joint meeting between representatives of the state health ministry and UNICEF.

At the meeting, it became clear that the federal government was finding it hard to accept anything about the project. They could not get over their concern about the fact that measles vaccine had never been used previously in India in any significant quantity. They repeatedly brought up the number of doses of vaccine—68,000—as if that in itself were a monstrous hurdle to overcome. They also expressed anxiety that no research had ever been carried out in India on measles vaccine.

I tried to set their minds at rest. "Well, doctor," I told the chief government spokesman, "if you like, when the vaccine arrives in Madras we will donate 2,000 doses of it to the federal government to use in a research project, in whatever manner you choose."

"At what cost, sir?" he responded.

"It will be our gift, sir, for scientific research," I told him, and with the acceptance of this proposition, the meeting ended.

Chapter 12

The final clearance was received from the government, and the Indian committee asked me to telex Whitby for a final shipping date. The following day, this message was received from Bill Nurse: "Bud Crookes advises vaccine going twentieth Air India. Number of flight to Madras will follow. Best wishes from today's Rotary meeting."

At last, it seemed to me that all was in order, but Krish, more knowledgeable about Indian bureaucracy, was less certain that our troubles were over. "Ken, we still have a long way to go. Even though the government has approved the shipment, they can just as easily change their minds."

He was right, but it was not what we had expected. Suddenly the tables were turned and the Indians had a laugh on me. Shortly after receiving the above telex regarding the date of shipment, I received a second telex from Bill Nurse. "Bud Crookes advises money delayed by bank. Shipment to go on September 22nd. Will advise flight number."

Throughout the previous days, I had constantly reassured my Indian friends that all would go as planned by Bud Crookes and Bill Nurse. Then, from out of nowhere, a foul-up occurred at the Canadian end. They had missed the deadline for getting the funds for the vaccine to Merck, Sharpe and Dohme. The saga of shipping difficulties was to continue. I telexed them on September 24, asking whether the measles vaccine had been shipped, and requesting that they advise us immediately of any delay. I received another telex from Whitby: "Long lateness story. Vaccine shipped Air India flight 104 (one-zero-four) Tuesday twenty-fifth, routed Bombay then Madras, flight I.C. 171 arrive Thursday night. Five-day ice pack—need repacking after arrival."

· Madras, September 1979 ·

The state government then demanded that we produce the air waybill with all the relevant details, and more telexes were exchanged with Bill Nurse. The most important one read: "Air billing number 12888654 leaves on September 25/79 06:20 Bombay flight 171. Arrives Thursday 20:35. Thirty-four containers, twenty-nine fiber cartons. Advise receipt of goods. Bill Nurse."

Following this telex, I received one from the manufacturer in New York:

> Measles vaccine of 34 containers and 29 fiber cartons weighing 3201 lb. For Rotary Club of Madras Charitable Trust will arrive by ICI 171 /28 Sep from Bom under customs BO DEEE BOND which is to be frozen immediately on AABAL EEE arrival. Grateful if you could arrange to get confirmation of arrival on this flight and to give necessary assistance at the airport for completion of formalities and transfer of this vaccine to M/S Spencer and Co. for necessary storage. Thanks. Representative of Rotary Club of Madras Charitable Trust will be at the airport on arrival for completion of formalities and to take delivery. Thanks for your cooperation and assistance.

Merck, Sharpe and Dohme followed the above telex with a cable. They obviously had very little faith in the Indian governmental system.

> Rahway N.J.—Urgent for action re: order 68,000 single doses Attenuvax measles virus vaccine live packed in 34 insulated containers weighing 2,890 lb. (85 lb. each) plus 29 fiber containers containing 68,000 vials 7ml sterile diluent 28, weighing 14 lbs. gross each and one weighing 5 lb. gross being shipped on Air India flight 104 AWB 12888654 ETD New York 1950 hours

> 25 September ETA Bombay 0620 hours September 27 transfer to flight 171 same day ETD 1900 hours Madras 2135 hours 27 September refrigerate vaccine immediately after arrival if material does not arrive as stated above notify us immediately: LAURIA MERCKRAH Telex 138825 33—67.

Our daily visits to various ministers at their offices continued. It became a ritual. At every government office we repeated the same phrases: "Measles is the most serious of all communicable diseases that can be prevented by immunization; measles causes more deaths than any other communicable disease that can be prevented by immunization; measles vaccine is safe; measles vaccine up until this time has never been available on a massive scale in India."

In each office I was reminded of the great patriot of India, Mahatma Gandhi, for in each ministerial office the Mahatma's Seven Social Sins, formulated in 1924, were displayed on the wall.

1. Politics without principle
2. Wealth without work
3. Commerce without morality
4. Education without character
5. Pleasure without conscience
6. Science without humanity
7. Worship without sacrifice

Over the years, I have noticed that Gandhi's list of sins has been silently removed from many Indian office walls. These seven sins are present in every society in the world. Perhaps a return to displaying them on the walls of the offices of all the world's politicians would help to restore our faith in society and upgrade our morality.

The next catastrophe was in the making. Twenty-four hours before the vaccine was to arrive in Bombay, a fire destroyed a large section of the

· Madras, September 1979 ·

cargo hangars in which we had planned to store it temporarily. All of us felt a deep concern for the safety of the vaccine, but we assumed that given its perishable nature it would be given priority in the cargo space that remained. Little was said and we went on our routine way preparing for the arrival of the vaccine in Madras at 9:15 p.m. on Friday evening, the 28th of September.

Krish and I sat in his office casually talking. The vaccine was to arrive in six hours' time. We chatted, laughing about the number of difficulties we had experienced. The most catastrophic was just a phone call away.

When the phone in his office rang, we both became instantly worried. As he spoke to the caller, Krish's smile vanished, and he appeared distressed. He placed the phone back on its cradle, summoned his secretary and hurriedly spoke to him in Tamil. He turned to me and said, "Let's go."

"Where?" I asked.

"Ken, just follow me. We have a major problem with the shipment."

As we drove towards one of the many government buildings we frequented, Krish told me that the state government had just denied permission to remove the vaccine, which was to arrive from Bombay in less than six hours now, from the tarmac. When we arrived in this large and now very familiar government office, we found it empty. We were on the eve of a state religious holiday. All government offices would be closed for four days.

Kumar, Gopal (whom I had nicknamed "Air France"), Krish and I were the only ones present. They were speaking in rapid-fire Tamil; I had learned a few words but nowhere near enough to follow this conversation. Quickly, they came to a decision, and Gopal, turning to me, said, "Come with me." I followed him to another room. Krish and Kumar departed in a different direction.

Gopal explained the situation to me. For some reason, the state government had decided, at the very last minute, not to allow the vaccine to be removed from the tarmac. And because of the religious holiday, it would be deposited there and left for four days unless we came up with a plan,

"That's incredible!" I exclaimed. "The vaccine has to be kept in freezer storage. They know that from the telex and cable from Merck. The vaccine will be destroyed if it sits in the sun for four days." I was on the verge of tears. We had spent two weeks constantly seeking agreement from the state government. Now it seemed that at the last moment we would once again be betrayed by government bureaucrats.

"This is India," Gopal answered. "I am sure we can solve the problem."

I looked around the large empty office, filled with an endless disarrangement of desks. There was only one beaten-up old typewriter for the whole place. Gopal excused himself and left the room. I sat down and waited, pondering. Why had I volunteered? Why I was in India? What I was attempting to do was for Rotary, and for the ideal of service above self. But was it even possible? I pondered the past several months, and found that I could no longer remember why I had volunteered in the first place. It was time to sort things out, and to attempt to put into clear perspective exactly what I was attempting to accomplish.

Quickly I reviewed my own personal goals of service. I knew why I had become involved in Rotary International, didn't I? Of course I did. I had always wanted to travel to faraway places. I had always wanted to help people in any way I could. Then I let my mind wander down several paths, finally settling on the reality of the present problem, and debating with myself whether it was or was not solvable.

I regained my composure, and told myself to concentrate on the matter at hand. I scanned the enormous office I was sitting in, and, my curiosity aroused, I began to wonder how many employees worked in this room with only one typewriter. Counting desks and work areas, I came up with the estimate of two hundred civil servants, all working together in this overrun office.

The walls were lined with tall, wooden file shelves, some six feet high, stacked up to the ceiling. There appeared to be literally miles of shelving, all loaded to capacity. Each storage area had a minimum of six shelves, and they appeared to be in a helter-skelter unorganized mess.

· Madras, September 1979 ·

Thick, dog-eared files, encased in typical brown legal-sized file covers, were bound with pieces of string or cotton bias tape in different colors: some red, some a dirt brown, others colorless. The file folders were stacked one on top of each other, rather than being stored horizontally. After thinking about the disarray, I came to the conclusion that the different colored ties probably indicated what the files contained. It did not seem like a particularly good system. These speculations occupied me for some time. Even now I marvel at how they ever retrieved the file they wanted. I was reminded of Krish's statement that the British had established disorganized bureaucracy in India, and the Indians had perfected it.

It was now 4:45 p.m. Gopal had been gone for more than an hour. I began to think that the next problem I would have to solve would be the question "Where are the others?" There was no sign of Gopal, Krish or Kumar. Had they forgotten where they had left me?

Suddenly, Gopal rushed into the room from the door on my left, with a person who turned out to be a secretary. At the same moment, Krish and Kumar appeared from the right, and all four of them converged on the desk with the archaic typewriter. Gopal and Kumar stood beside the secretary, who seated himself at the machine and prepared to type. Krish approached me, and sat down.

"Ken," he said, "we have a temporary solution. I phoned Delhi and talked with the minister. Then we contacted the chief minister's office here in Madras. We have been given permission to remove the vaccine from the airport and take it to Spencer's for cold storage. But we will not be permitted to open or unpack the containers."

"But, Krish," I protested, "we must open the containers when we get them to the freezer. The containers act as insulators; if we don't remove the vaccine the cold will not be able to contact the vaccine. It may become unusable. Its potency will deteriorate."

Krish, of course, knew all this as well as I did. "Ken," he said, "we will cross that road tomorrow. At least we have the vaccine under our control, for the time being at least."

This was the best we could do, apparently. I resigned myself to the situation, hoping that for one more night the vaccine would remain viable and potent.

At 9:30 p.m. on Friday, September 28, as Air India flight 171 from Bombay arrived in Madras with no fanfare or publicity, history was made. Krish, Kumar, President C.T., Gopal, Eva and I stood in the cargo area of the Madras airport as the trolleyload of vaccine was brought to the unloading area. This was first time that measles vaccine in any significant volume had ever landed in India. What was perhaps more important, the fact that the vaccine had arrived duty-free, and had been shipped free of charge by Air India, signaled a dramatic change in Indian public health and the expanded program of immunization (EPI).

The vaccine was quickly loaded on the trucks that C.T. had donated from his business. The vaccine was then taken immediately to Spencer's walk-in freezers. I wanted to open and unpack all of the containers, but I realized that this could place the entire project in jeopardy. One container, however, was opened and the freezer packs were found to be still frozen solid. This was reassuring; I felt that all would be in order overnight.

As we sat in the dining room of the Connemara Hotel enjoying a gin and tonic (purchased courtesy of C.T.'s liquor permit), a feeling of accomplishment was enjoyed by all. The day we had all worked so hard for had come and gone. We could not know then what far-reaching changes our efforts would produce for all of the children of India.

Chapter 13

The next morning, while we were at breakfast, the phone rang. Krish spoke to the caller for a few minutes in a low voice and then abruptly hung up. He looked at me with a smile and said, "Ken, this morning you are going to see the real India. Kumar's secretary will be here in fifteen minutes to take you and Eva to another government office to straighten out the problem with the vaccine. Unfortunately, you will have to do this by yourselves, as both Kumar and I have other commitments."

The driver arrived, and we left at once. After a ten-minute drive from Krish's house, we pulled up outside a rundown old two-storey house, which was used as a government office. The sign on the building read "Director of Civil Supply."

I glanced at my watch as we climbed the outside staircase; it was 9:15 a.m. At the top of the stairs there was a large crowd sitting on the floor and standing against the pillars. We followed the secretary into the office, and he announced our arrival.

We were quickly ushered into the director's inner office. What a shock! A small man sat huddled over a small filthy desk. Numerous papers were strewn at random on top of this antiquated piece of furniture. To his right, on a small stand, was a telephone that appeared to have a padlock on the rotary dial. Fortunately, the windows were open, allowing a breeze to pass from one side of the office to the other. This minimal air circulation helped to dispel the odor of the room. The director motioned us to be seated, and while we waited I took a more careful look around the room. I observed, to my amazement, that the floor and the furniture were fouled with a multitude of bird droppings. The director was busily engaged with a young woman, who was attempting to increase her free supply of kerosene. Kumar's secretary, who had accompanied us, translated for me. My first thought was "What in the world can this office have to do with our measles vaccine which arrived last evening?"

For the next hour, we listened to several Indians asking for increases in their present quotas of supplies. Every now and then an employee would knock on the window. The director would pause, unlock the phone, beckon the employee to come in, talk with him and then have him sign a register book, after which the employee would disappear outside again, and the director would pass the phone out to him through an opening that reminded me of the milk chute we had had at home when I was a youngster.

When the phone conversation was over, the procedure was repeated in reverse. The employee would pass the phone in through the opening, walk into the room through the door, sign the register, and depart. The director would then check the register, lock the phone and carry on his conversation with the individual he had been occupied with before this interruption.

Eva and I sat and smiled incredulously at each other. All of a sudden a bird flew in through an open window, landed on the director's desk and relieved itself on a piece of his correspondence. The director quickly and automatically cleared the document with his hand, carrying on his conversation as though nothing had happened. We could hardly contain ourselves.

I glanced at my watch. It was now 10:45 a.m. I whispered to Kumar's secretary, "When are we going to be able to speak with the director?"

"I don't know," he replied.

My frustration level became more severe. The little drama of unlocking and re-locking the phone happened at least once every ten minutes. The birds continued to fly in and out of the windows. Our reflex to duck was now well conditioned. People were petitioning for more petrol, kerosene, propane, fertilizer, and other farm products. My mind wandered back to our measles vaccine, which was waiting to be unpacked in the walk-in freezers of Spencer's store. I failed to understand what this funny little man could possibly have to do with it.

I heard a clock outside chime twelve noon; and I became even more anxious. We had now been sitting in front of the director's desk for almost three hours, and not a word had been addressed to us. I had tried to negotiate an opening of conversation on several occasions, but was always met with a blank stare from the director.

Kumar's secretary had on several occasions excused himself and left the room for fifteen or twenty minutes. As the chimes of noon died away, he re-entered and I beckoned to him. He leaned over and I said in a low tone into his ear: "My wife and I are leaving at 12:30. We are going to Spencer's to uncrate the containers. They can throw me in jail if they like. I have sat here long enough. I know that the store will be closing at 1:30 p.m. for the holiday and I am not going to wait that long."

He seemed alarmed. "You can't do that," he whispered anxiously, "I have instructions from Mr. Kumar to stay here till we talk with the director."

I ignored him. I leaned over and told Eva that we would be leaving shortly and to follow me. At precisely 12:30 p.m. I stood up and left the room. The director, who was involved in a bitter conversation with a disgruntled farmer, appeared not to notice.

We dashed down the stairs and ran to the nearby corner, where we hailed a three-wheeled taxi to take us to Spencer's. The traffic was heavy and I kept my eyes on my watch. When the taxi finally rolled up at Spencer's door, it was 1:15 p.m.

It took me several minutes to find the person in charge of the freezers. When I told him I wanted to enter the one where the vaccine was stored, he quickly asked, "Who is going to help you?"

"My wife," I replied.

He seemed to understand from my tone that I meant what I said, and without any argument he ushered us out the back door of the store and opened the freezer locker. It was indeed cold in the freezer. The outside temperature was 40 degrees Celsius (104 degrees Fahrenheit), and approximately 100 percent humidity; inside, the weather was arctic.

With Eva's help, I started opening and unloading the thirty-four containers of vaccine. Each container held 2000 doses in individual vials. I was relieved to see that the storage packs in the containers were still frozen solid.

Despite the cold, we continued with the job. When we had half of the containers unloaded, Krish arrived. "Ken," he protested, "you can't do this. We do not have permission from the director of civil supplies."

"They can put me in jail for all I care," I answered. Krish, who had seemed angry when he arrived, now began to help, and the work progressed rapidly. We opened each container, checked the contents, and unpacked the vials of vaccine and placed them on the shelves. Then we carried the empty containers to the outer storage area. We were on the last container when I heard a new and distinctive Indian voice behind me.

"You are very impatient, sir. You must remember you are in India, and here we go by the rules. You must respect the law."

I turned around and there stood the director of civil supplies.

"Fine," I said, pointing to the shelves, "We have unpacked 64,000 doses of measles vaccine. If you wish to count them, go ahead."

"No, sir," he said, "it is too cold—I will take your word—but please, in the future, be a little more patient with us." With that he departed, and we never encountered that particular gentleman again.

Chapter 14

My major assignment was now complete. The vaccine had arrived and was stored in a safe, reliable, refrigerated environment. Eva and I had another six days in Madras before we were to resume the round-the-world trip we had planned to celebrate our twenty-fifth wedding anniversary.

Our last few nights in Madras were spent as our previous evenings had been, visiting close friends of Susheila and Krish Chitale's. I was overwhelmed by the kindness of the South Indians. Even on first meeting they had an uncanny ability to make you feel very comfortable and at home; it was as if they had known you for eons.

We spent one of our remaining evenings at President C.T. and Seeta's home; it was a very memorable occasion. Seeta's warmth and pleasant smile will always be with us. A deep friendship had been established, one that still thrives today, after some twenty-one years.

Talking with Krish's friends on those pleasant evenings, I came to the unavoidable realization that all the problems were not solved. The 68,000 doses of measles vaccine that we had contributed were only a drop in the bucket. The city of Madras had a population of over five million: only a few tens of thousands among them would be vaccinated. We had won a battle; but the disease was still winning the war. I knew now that not all Rotarians were as service-motivated as Krish or myself. Some of the Rotarian medical doctors I had met had attitudes that I found perplexing—they were angry that we were infringing on their ability to make a living. The thought of these doctors and their selfish concerns nagged at me, though I tried to put them out of my mind. I was reminded of them on several occasions when we were discussing the outcome of the project.

As we climbed the stairway to board the Indian Airlines flight to New Delhi, I turned and waved to Krish and Susheila. After we were seated, I turned to Eva and said, "I have the feeling we'll be back in Madras in the near future."

As the plane took off, our conversation was interrupted by the noise of the engines and the safety announcements by the stewardess. When we were in the air and cabin was quieter, Eva turned to me and asked, "Why did you say that? What makes you think that we will be back?"

"It's just an inner feeling that I have. We have only scratched the surface of what needs to be done. There are so many needs and so little time to help. That's why I said we will back soon."

My prophetic thoughts would be proved right many times over the next twenty-one years.

Our three-day stay in New Delhi at the Maurya Sheraton Hotel was very relaxing. On the second day we took a tour of the city by taxi, with a most helpful driver. He suggested that we take the triangular tour to Agra-Jaipur-New Delhi over a four-day period. The cost was 1200 rupees ($400 Canadian). The following morning we were picked up at the hotel by our taxi driver.

Our trip to Agra was interspersed with visits to other temples. Our first glimpse of the Taj Mahal was unforgettable, and our guide, seeing how moved we were by the beauty of this extraordinary edifice, offered to take us back to see it again at dusk, and at sun-up the following morning. We declined, but with appreciative thanks.

Our drive to Jaipur was long, slow and tiring. When we had to wait at a train crossing, the driver stopped the car and beckoned us to follow him into a local home at the side of the road. It was a mud hut, with an earthen floor. The outside was painted with cow dung and cow's urine, and inside, the floor was covered with a cow-dung paste. The driver told us that the dung had two important properties: first, it sanitized the floor, and second, it kept the dust under control. The lady of the house was

Madras, September 1979

cooking breakfast over her open dung-fired stove. She offered some of her *chapati*, which we turned down as graciously as we could.

The driver gave as a short history of the area and we stopped a multitude of times to visit ancient temples and palaces. The most spectacular was the Fortress of the Winds, which was built on a very high hill. The Maharajah who had built it did not take into account the shortage of water in the area. Consequently the life span of his fort-palace was short.

In the Red City of Jaipur we stayed at the old Maharajah's palace. Our room was enormous. Even the bathroom was some twenty by twenty-five feet in size. The ceilings were covered with large salamanders at night.

Before leaving for Delhi the following morning, we visited several local carpet makers. I had been told of child labour being used in the hand-manufacture of Indian carpets. The children were used because their small hands were able to create a better product. I hesitated before ordering a custom-made twelve- by sixteen-foot wool and Dacron carpet. I compromised with my worried conscience, reasoning that if these children did not work, they would not eat; often they are the main breadwinners for themselves and younger brothers and sisters. The ethics of this question are still controversial.

Shortly after our arrival back in New Delhi, we were off again, flying to Hong Kong, where we were to join a small tour group to visit Thailand, Malaysia and Singapore.

At the end of the tour we visited Manila, where I had the opportunity of meeting a Rotarian acquaintance, a former group study exchange leader. Bernie Hernandez from the Philippines had visited our district the previous year; we were pleased when he flew up from the southern island of Mindanao to be with us for the weekend. Through him, Eva and I met a Rotarian we will always cherish and respect, Dr. Benny Santos.

It was by coincidence that we met Dr. Benny. Bernie had invited Eva and me to accompany him to the home of a fellow Rotarian for a drink, and our host asked us if we would like to attend a Rotary meeting. Of course we were happy to, and we set off to the club's meeting place, a large hall outside Manila. The atmosphere was very quiet and disciplined. However, halfway through the noon-hour meeting, a small, smiling, and very energetic Rotarian entered in a rush, and the effect was as if someone had set off a bomb. The feeling in the hall was completely changed, all because of the powerful, contagious personality of Dr. Benny Santos.

After the meeting Benny asked Eva and me to come next door to his office, because he was eager to hear more about our activities in India, which he had heard about from other members of the club. On entering his office I was amazed to see some fifty or sixty patients waiting for his return. Benny ushered us into his large open consulting room, seated us in front of his desk and introduced us to his wife, who also acted as his office manager. She too had desk space in the consulting room.

Benny and I talked about Rotary, and about Rotary in India in particular. After ten minutes, beginning to feel uncomfortable, I reminded him that there were a lot of patients waiting for his expertise.

He brushed my concern aside." They will wait. You see, Ken, my fees are very affordable—they will wait! I can see my patients tomorrow, but I cannot talk about Rotary with you tomorrow because you will be gone. So let's continue! Rotary is such a good organization, and we both love it so."

Ten minutes later his wife once again approached Benny and in Spanish reminded him of the number of patients waiting. He ignored her and went on talking. After forty-five minutes I was at last able to persuade him that we had to leave, and we rose to take our departure and let him get back to work. He reluctantly agreed, but insisted that we take a group photo on the steps of his office building. After the picture-taking we left.

Our paths have crossed many times since that memorable afternoon. Benny is still the kind-hearted, joyful, and enthusiastically committed Rotarian that he was on that Saturday outside Manila in October 1979.

After a brief stay in Fiji, we returned home to Whitby.

We had been gone nine weeks. The two months had gone extremely fast but they were not soon to be forgotten. Our experiences in India had made an indelible impression. The rest of the world was still just names on a map, but India was inscribed in large capital letters.

The district governor had asked a member of our club, Bill Irwin, to hold a meeting with another past district governor to discuss the possibility of expanding the program under a Rotary International 3H grant. (The name 3H stands for health, hunger and humanity. This program was launched by Rotary International President Clem Renouf of Australia. He asked every Rotarian in the world to donate a minimum of $15 (US) as a birthday gift to Rotary on its seventy-fifth birthday. He had hoped to raise some $13 (US) million to be used in the developing world. Unfortunately, only $9 million plus was raised, but this started the 3H Program, which is still in existence today.)

When Bill Irwin asked me if I would help with this new initiative, my reply was short and simple. I will contact Rotarian Krish Chitale, I told them, and if he is in agreement then we can proceed. Once again, Rotarian Bill Nurse provided, free of charge, the telex network. The following telex was sent on November 7, 1979:

> Gov. Paul suggests that we explore the possibility of a 3H project in 1980 to provide Rotary District 320 a minimum of 1/2 million doses of Attenuvax. It would be in multiple shipments. We require your approval before November the 13th in order to start long process here. Detailed letter to follow. Signed, Ken Hobbs, M.D.

On the November 12, 1979, a reply was received from Krish, which read:

> Thank you for yr tlx of Nov. 7. Extremely pleased to accept yr district's generous offer of half a million doses of vaccine. Discussed with health Secretary and obtained

clearance from state govt. Will make other necessary applications after receipt of yr detailed letter. Please convey our thanks to Governor Paul and other fellow Rtns. Special regards and thanks from Governor Venu, President C.T. and the Rtns of Madras. Signed, Krish.

The mechanism to proceed was now in place.

I had not anticipated at that moment in December 1979 that I would be visiting India thirteen times over the next fifteen years, or that twelve of these trips would be at no cost to the project or to Rotary International. The other members of the committee visited India twice each, once in "phase one" and once in "phase two." The cost of these visits would be included in the project's budget. Four other non-committee volunteers would experience a visit to South India to monitor the project, and their costs were also included in the budget of the project. The only visit that was included in either phase one or phase two for my personal air travel expenses was my visit in 1984. The money for my airfare was donated back to The Rotary Foundation. The reason for the apparent oversight of not including expenses for a visit by the treasurer in phase two is open for speculation. Eva's and my visits have always been personally financed.

A committee was formed to administer the 3H and CIDA grants. This was composed of the present district governor, Paul McKelvey of Alliston, the incoming district governor, Fran Smith of Scarborough, the incoming district governor after Fran Smith, Fred Black of Guelph, Past District Governor Wilf Wilkinson of Trenton, and myself, as a non-office-holding Rotarian. My role was to act as medical consultant and supervise the implementation of the project. Governor Paul acted as chairman, and Past District Governor Wilf Wilkinson as treasurer.

The role of "medical consultant" was vague. However, I interpreted the role as gofer and doer. I realized that by voluntarily taking on extra responsibilities, I was leaving myself open to criticism, some of which I would receive publicly, and some of which would be voiced quietly, behind the scenes. I challenged myself to overlook their insecurities in these concerns.

However, I have never understood or concerned myself with the pecking order in our Rotary District, or at Rotary International. I was prepared to do what needed to be done in order to make this a successful venture. I had committed myself to persuading the Indian government to make measles vaccination a priority, and I would only consider my job to be finished when measles became a part of their EPI program. (EPI stands for "expanded program for immunization.") In 1979, this was still a long way down the road (it was finally accepted as part of their EPI program in 1985). My second objective was to attempt to ensure that someday all vaccines would be manufactured in India itself, instead of having to be imported. Unfortunately, time did not allow this personal priority of mine ever to become a reality, though I pursued it rather intensely.

The requirements for the Indians' participation in the expanded program were outlined in a letter from me to Krish on the December 4, 1979, and were as follows: 1. The Indian minister of health must sign a "hold harmless" agreement to the effect that any legal implications were the responsibility of the Indian government and not Rotary International. The agreement was drawn up by Rotary International. (This was essential before any 3H funding could be approved.) 2. An agreement had to be secured from World Health Organization. 3. The project organizers must inform the committee of the number of children under the age of five years in the states of Tamil Nadu and Kerala. 4. They must also obtain accurate information of the number of children who had died from measles and its complications in South India in each of the previous two years. A letter was sent to Dr. Ralph Henderson at WHO in Geneva, thanking him for his assistance and intervention in September 1979, without which the project could not have been started, let alone successfully completed. He replied:

> Thank you for your letter of December the 4th 1979. We are happy to have been of assistance in facilitating the

exchange of information between Rotary Clubs and Government of India. However, I would like to stress that, although we are very sympathetic to the measles immunization program organized by Rotary Clubs in Southern India, we are not in a position to formally approve or endorse it. Such approval may be issued only by the Director General of Health Services of the Government of India, which coordinates various activities of the existing and planned immunization programs. The EPI section of this health service organizes the immunization services, works on the expansion of immunization coverage of eligible infants, and keeps liaison with international agencies on technical matters. I would therefore advise you to contact Dr. N. Basu, assistant director general of health services, EPI, Nirman Bhavan, New Delhi.

If I can be of any further assistance, however, please do not hesitate to contact us. Dr. Ralph Henderson, Director, Expanded Program on Immunization.

The year 1979 came to a close with a satisfying sense of some viable accomplishment, however small.

Chapter 15

The New Year, 1980, started quietly, in the usual manner. However, it would soon be interrupted by the constant intrusion of problems with the measles vaccine program. I could not know that 1980 would be as difficult as 1979 and at times much more arduous.

Communications with Krish became a weekly or biweekly routine: letters, telexes, sometimes, in desperation, even a phone call. Placing a phone call was an onerous task (as I mentioned in Chapter 3): you had to go through long distance operators in Montreal, then London, then Bombay. Only at the end of this relay of operators would you at last be connected with the operator in Madras.

Voice transmission was difficult. The inability to hear the faint voice in the background made one feel one had to yell, which meant that both parties had great difficulty in understanding what was being said. Telephone calls were made only as a last resort.

Our list of problems to be solved boiled down to three essential areas of concern.

First and foremost was the need to get the governments of the states of Tamil Nadu and Kerala to sign a "hold harmless" agreement. This, from Rotary International's point of view, was mandatory. They would not even consider our proposal, much less release money for the proposed project, unless we could provide such an agreement, releasing Rotary International of any legal implications in this or any other project receiving funding from The Rotary Foundation.

Second, I was still pursuing the Indian government to pay for the cost of the air freight for the original shipment of 68,000 doses of measles vaccine. Merck, Sharpe and Dohme had paid for the air transport rather than hold up the shipment in September. The mix-up had been due to a difference of opinion over who should have been responsible for this.

Third, the statistics regarding measles had still not been supplied to us. We needed to know the population of children under the age of five in South India; the morbidity and mortality rate of red measles or measles; sequelae of the disease and other factors. This information was indispensable to our attempt to persuade the 3H committee to approve our program of immunizing 3.5 million children of the states of Tamil Nadu and Kerala against red measles.

I wrote Dr. N. Basu, the assistant director general of health services for the Expanded Program of Immunization in New Delhi. I explained to him the need for the federal government's intervention, in order to approve the cost of the shipment by Air India in September in the amount of $7,237.78 (Cdn). I also enclosed a copy of Rotary International's "hold harmless" agreement, for his information. I explained our plan to apply for a 3.5-million-dose program of measles immunization for South India. This project would cost approximately $500,000 (US), and was conditional upon the signing of the agreement.

It was not until late April that I recognized that health services, including immunization, were a state responsibility, and that therefore the federal government was not the level of government that I should be pursuing in regard to the agreement. This detail would prove to be a stumbling block as far as Rotary International was concerned. Fortunately, in early May I was able to convince John Stucky, the manager of Rotary International's 3H program, that immunization was indeed a state responsibility. I further convinced him that Rotary International should honor and accept the "hold harmless" agreements signed by the two states, Tamil Nadu and Kerala.

Krish needed to know the exact number of doses we would require, so that he could apply to the Ministry of Civil Aviation and Tourism for free air transportation of the vaccine by Air India from New York to Madras. I

·January – April 1980·

appreciated that once they approved a certain number, they would be loath to change the amount. I explained that the number of doses would be contingent upon our final application and the finalizing of the cost per dose. We had not as yet established a guaranteed price with the manufacturer, Merck, Sharpe and Dohme. Early in the exchange of information with Krish, I had established a minimum of two million doses of vaccine. On February 9, 1980, Krish forwarded me a copy of a letter which he had sent to Dr. Ranjit Sen, director general of the health services of India in New Delhi. He outlined our initial 68,000-dose program and described our proposal to enlarge the scope of the measles immunization program. He requested that Dr. Ranjit Sen, with the Minister of Civil Aviation, issue an affidavit for free air transport of at least six shipments of 500,000 doses each from New York to Madras. The exact dimensions and weights would be known in the near future.

Interspersed with these problems was a continuing lack of cooperation from the medical doctors of Tamil Nadu. Krish forwarded me a copy of a letter to the editor of the *Indian Express* newspaper by Dr. Jacob John (of the Christian Medical College in Madras), who had had this to say:

> In response to the various letters appearing in the press recently, I would like to clarify several erroneous statements, firstly, the experience with the live attenuated measles virus vaccine (Attenuvax) in the United States has been entirely happy. The unpleasant experience referred to in the letters was in relation to another vaccine, namely the inactivated (killed) measles virus vaccine, which has not been used for over twelve years.
>
> Secondly, Attenuvax does not "cause fever with rash almost as severe as naturally acquired measles." It causes no fever at all in over 90 percent of children. Mild or moderate fever for one or two days may occur in fewer than 10 percent of children between the seventh and the

tenth day after immunization. Children with these reactions continue to play, and are not sick, unlike children with measles who become miserable and very sick. Moreover, the other symptoms of measles: namely conjunctivitis, rhinitis, cough, Koplick's spots, sore mouths, diarrhea, etc. are totally absent in vaccinated children. All complications of measles are also totally absent. These, then are the advantages of measles immunization.

Thirdly, a number of vaccination trials have already been conducted in India using the live measles vaccine. These reports are available in the various medical journals. All trials have been entirely satisfactory, indicating the absolute safety and the extreme efficacy of this vaccine in India. In the last three months we have immunized over nine thousand children in Vellore and nearby villages, without any serious reactions.

Let me make a plea to my professional colleagues to refrain from misinforming the public. All technical and scientific information are available through the usual scientific media. I shall be happy to answer directly and personally any further specific questions that any of your readers might have.

Dr. T. Jacob John, Professor and Head,
Department of Virology, C.M.C Hospital, Vellore.

I received the above press clipping from Dr. Jacob John in a letter dated February 28, 1980. Here are excerpts from his letter:

> We now have used up 11,000 doses and have a clinic this afternoon which will exhaust our 12,000 doses...after bringing the vaccine I have tested the potency of the vaccine. To my happy surprise the potency is 5000 TCID 50

per dose. The company need not have included more than 3200 TCID50, and I suspect that they took extra caution in preparing it for India.... I trust you had a pleasant time in India. We will be looking forward to your next visit. You, almost single-handedly, have changed the course of history in Southern India in the field of public health.

I had accepted the challenge of John Stucky, Rotary International Director of the Health, Hunger and Humanity Program to be the second worldwide volunteer to work in a Vietnamese refugee camp in Hong Kong in March-April 1980.

This was indeed a pleasant surprise. I was to be the second volunteer in a boat camp in Hong Kong. Rotary International would pay my airfare and give me $200 weekly to pay for our room at the YMCA in Hong Kong. Eva's airfare was our own expense. (So Rotary International got two for the price of one.)

We left home the end of February. We arrived at the airport in Hong Kong at 11:30 p.m. after a twelve-hour flight. We were astounded when we were paged and informed that we were being met by Dr. Dale and Dr. Wong. Dr. Dale was head of the camp and the Hong Kong Christian Mission.

Dr. Wong was from Montreal, and was formerly from South Vietnam. He had arrived in Hong Kong three days prior to our arrival. If I was ever to be second to anyone, thank God it was Dr. Wong. He was a quiet, gentle, humble man, who showed us around downtown Kowloon the following morning. He pointed out the post office, the bank, the bus area where we would catch our bus, where we could find good value for our money— the best shopping, restaurants, etc. He introduced us to *dim sum* for lunch. Our next eight weeks would be full of excitement and new experiences.

Our regular routine Monday to Friday was soon etched in stone. We would awaken at 6:00 a.m., go for breakfast behind the old YMCA. Catch the bus for the Jubilee and Samshuipo refugee camps at ten minutes to seven. On the bus, the next forty-five minutes would be spent observing all the sights and sounds and smells of the old back streets of Hong Kong.

Butchers were killing their ducks and chickens on the curb in front of their cramped premises on the narrow back streets. Elderly men would be transporting freshly roasted pigs strapped to the bar of their bicycles, with the front legs tied neatly beneath their handlebars, and the rear legs tied methodically below their seat. They had the knack of straddling the cooked pig with grace as they pedaled down the narrow busy streets.

Local men and women were having coffee and breakfast at the crowded little street hovels that served as restaurants. On every piece of open ground seniors were doing *tai chi*. Every now and then we would observe a group of men playing a game that involved gambling, and becoming quite heated and vociferous at times.

Others carried bird cages. From time to time we would pass a solitary tree and there would be several men settled under it with their bird cages. It seemed, from their conversations and gestures, that they were comparing the attributes and beauty of their various species of birds. Every day on our trip through Hong Kong we were treated to different sights, sounds and dramas. We always looked forward to this early-morning adventure on the back streets of the city.

On entering the camp, we were greeted by the camp security guards. They would give us a broad smile and say something, which we never caught, in Chinese.

The medical center was close by. The nurses were English and well trained. This was my first experience practicing medicine through an interpreter. After a short time I managed to pick up a few common Vietnamese medical phrases.

Eva was put to work in the small pharmacy. She did whatever the nurses asked: dispensing, sewing, packaging. As a matter of fact, after two days dispensing various antibiotics, she had learned enough to start questioning my judgment. The nurses then asked if she too was a nurse. "No," I told them, "she's just an all-round expert."

· January – April 1980 ·

We worked at the Samshuipo camp in the morning. It was an old British army camp, which had been used as a prison camp by the Japanese after the fall of Hong Kong in December 1942. I would see approximately 125 patients every morning and another 125 at sick bay at the Jubilee Transit Center in the afternoon. It was busy and demanding; hard work, but very gratifying and enjoyable.

There were approximately 15,000 residents. The refugees were housed in the old buildings. Each family had a bunk measuring approximately six by eight feet, and a family of four would live, with all of their personal possessions, in this small space. The bunks were three tiers high, with a narrow isle between the tiers.

The residents would cook on gas-fired woks. A covered, communal eating area was set aside. The method of cooking, plus the crowded conditions, produced a large number of second-degree burns on the children.

They were assigned to a toilet and issued a key to the facility. In the morning there would be lineups at the toilets, which stood side by side in a row that stretched a considerable distance. The camp bordered on the ocean with a high steel fence. The children would play various games and occupy their time outdoors. An old double-decker bus had been converted into a play area. It was a pleasure to observe the children playing so harmoniously.

The crowded living conditions produced coughs, bronchitis, and other upper-respiratory-tract infections. There were also some outbreaks of scabies, a contagious skin disease characterized by intense itching. Eva became very familiar with this condition, and expert at treating it. Shampooing and bathing children who suffered from scabies came instinctively to her. Every day she gently cared for at least thirty children. On her last day, the nurses presented her with a diploma certifying that she was a registered "scabies technician." This diploma now hangs in our office at home.

The afternoons were spent next door at the Jubilee Transit Camp. Our routine there was the same. At 4:30 p.m. we would get back on the bus.

The forty-five-minute return journey was always interesting. The smells, sounds and experiences were totally different in the afternoon, on our way back to the YMCA, than they had been in the morning. We will always remember our happy days with these cheerful refugees.

The first few days we considered repainting our room and bathroom on the fifth floor of the YMCA (this was direly needed). We were met every evening as we left the elevator by our floor man. I soon trained him to bring me an insulated container of ice, which I purchased for one Hong Kong dollar (twenty-five cents Canadian). I can honestly say that I was surely the only person in the YMCA having ice in my Scotch those evenings.

After several more days of cleaning and reorganizing, our room became very appealing. We had a good TV, and our window opened on the side of the Peninsular Hotel. It was very pleasant to be so close. They had an excellent deli, where we would sometimes shop for a quick supper. Other evenings, we would walk into the back streets and pick a restaurant. We wanted to be off the regular tourist route. We would pick only those with a menu written in Chinese. We would pick our entrees by pointing to an item. This form of Russian roulette was usually very satisfactory. Most of the time we were both happy and surprised by our choices.

The weekends were our days off. I worked every other Saturday morning, leaving Eva to rest in bed. We would shop on Saturday afternoons, and on Sunday we would ride the double-decker trolley buses around the island and up to the new territories. After eight weeks we became very familiar with Hong Kong.

Before we left for Hong Kong in late February, I had notified Krish that we would be staying at the YMCA in Kowloon. In mid-February I had submitted a preliminary 3H application for our expanded red measles program in South India to John Stucky. The total budget called for in the preliminary application was $375,100 (US), which provided for 3.5 million doses of measles vaccine in multiple-dose vials of fifty doses per vial.

In Hong Kong, I was still deeply involved in corresponding with

· January – April 1980 ·

Krish via letter and cable. In one communication he informed me that the final 68,000 doses had been distributed as follows:

> Institute of Child Health, Madras .... 12,000 doses
> C.M.C., Vellore .... 12,000 doses
> Railway Hospital, Perambur, Madras ..... 2,000 doses
> Coimbatore Clubs .... 12,000 doses
> Tanjore Club .... 4,000 doses
> C.M.C Hospital [second installment] ..... 12,000 doses
> State of Kerala .... 14,000 doses
> **Total** .... 68,000 doses

In another letter, Krish forwarded the statistics required for Rotary International:

> The number of births for the first half of this decade are predicted as follows:
>
> | | | |
> |---|---|---|
> | 1980 | 1.74 million | 1.566 million will survive |
> | 1981 | 1.77 million | 1.593 million will survive |
> | 1982 | 1.80 million | 1.620 million will survive |
> | 1983 | 1.83 million | 1.647 million will survive |
> | 1984 | 1.83 million | 1.674 million will survive |
>
> Deaths due to measles cannot be calculated with too much accuracy. In the northern parts of India, the official figure are six deaths per 1000 children with measles. In our experience in Tamil Nadu, we can expect death ranges up to 140 per 1000 with measles. To be very conservative I shall accept ten deaths per 1000 children. Calculated thus, the number of deaths among the surviving infants in Tamil Nadu would be as follows:
>
> 1980   17,400 anticipated deaths from measles under the age of 3

1981	17,700 anticipated deaths from measles under the age of 3
1982	18,000 anticipated deaths from measles under the age of 3
1983	18,300 anticipated deaths from measles under the age of 3
1984	18,600 anticipated deaths from measles under the age of 3

Dr. K.P.B. Nair of Trichur, Kerala, states that the 1971 census in the state showed that the number of children under the age of five constituted 14 percent of the total population of 21,347,375. Therefore there would be approximately 3,500,000 under the age of five in Kerala. After the epidemic of measles that was spreading across the state in February and March 1980, it is estimated that 40 percent would now be immune to red measles by the spring of 1980.

In early April, Krish wrote to inform me that he had met with the minister of health for the state of Tamil Nadu. The minister was in agreement with the "hold harmless" agreement that was required by Rotary International. However, he wanted to add a stipulation in the agreement that the state government would have the right to sue the manufacturer if any catastrophes occurred. This would prove to be a stumbling block for Rotary International, and John Stucky in particular, for the next three months. I forwarded a copy of Krish's letter to John Stucky for advisement. He replied to Krish that the board would not accept any variance from the original "hold harmless" agreement. Finally, three months later, the state government agreed to omit this clause. John Stucky informed Krish by telex on April 18, 1980:

> Our hold harmless agreement is between R.I. and ministry of health of India. We cannot contract to bind a third party. Suggest ministry of health seek a separate indemnity from supplier and quantity. You will have

opportunity prior to date of dispatch to refuse acceptance. Advice of ministry's acceptance of hold harmless agreement is needed prior to 3H committee meeting, May 5. Signed, John Stucky, 3H Manager.

Once again the pot was on the boil. My paramount responsibility was to inform John Stucky that it was the states of Tamil Nadu and Kerala, not the federal ministry of health, that had to sign the hold harmless agreement. It was confusing to him; as an American, he tended to assume that the responsibility rested with the federal government. This was not so.

The long road to correcting this aberration was arduous indeed. However, I finally overcame the reluctance on the part of Rotary International, and they accepted the hold harmless agreement signed by the two state health ministries some three months later.

On our arrival home after seven weeks in Hong Kong, a telex from Krish was waiting for me:

> Deep regret unable to proceed due to elections in a few states in India including Tamil Nadu. May not be able to receive signed hold harmless agreements till June. I have received oral confirmation of agreement from states of Tamil Nadu and Kerala dists 320 and 321 will proceed as of tlx 18th April of John Stucky. Regards, Chitale.

This telex was relayed to John Stucky on May 5. In a few days' time I received word from John Stucky that the project had been approved, conditional upon the signing of hold harmless agreements and free transportation of the vaccine from New York to Madras. Definite confirmation would be coming in a few weeks time.

As noted in Chapter 14, a committee to organize the project was formed by Governor Paul McKelvey of Alliston, consisting of himself as chairman, incoming governor Fran Smith of Scarborough, district governor nominee Fred Black of Guelph, who would follow Fran Smith as district governor, Past District Governor Wilf Wilkinson of Trenton, and myself. Wilf was asked to be treasurer, as his vocation was that of an accountant. Governor Paul had asked that I be the medical adviser and medical consultant for the project. The reason for this request was self-explanatory: no one else had any detailed knowledge of the preliminary project or indeed any knowledge of measles. The first meeting of the committee was called for August 18 at our home; the agenda was lunch and then an organizational meeting for the proposed project.

I soon realized that my role would be essential if this project was to succeed and stretch into a "phase two." In the end, the final phase would be wrapped up by the treasurer twelve years later, in 1992, without my ever being notified, although I had served as the medical director of the program. A proper final report by our committee was never submitted, nor was the idea of writing one ever entertained, even though I had spent considerable time in Madras in May 1993 collecting information for a final, thorough report. The cost of my visit in 1993 had been placed in the budget. I would have re-donated the airfare to The Rotary Foundation as I had in phase one. However, phase two would conclude suddenly without a comprehensive report or medical evaluation being accomplished. In my opinion, a final report was necessary and important. The committee's thirteen years of dedication to this important humanitarian endeavor would conclude suddenly, unexpectedly and unannounced.

Chapter 16

The management committee for the new 3H measles program in South India was approved at our District Assembly in April 1980. As the approval was being passed I quietly reminisced about the previous year, when I was a committee of one attempting to introduce red measles vaccine into India.

The resolution passed unanimously. I was hopeful that the expanded membership of the committee would make the task easier. I presumed that the change would mean there would be extra help, but even so, I realized that it would be up to Krish Chitale and myself to make the proposed project successful. No matter how big the committee grew, I knew that the real responsibility would still come back to the two of us.

My first task was to inform the committee of what had transpired on my initial visit to South India in September 1979, but I was cognizant of the fact that it would be difficult to convey to a group that knew nothing about India the true nature of the problems that I had encountered, or the imposing problems that still lay ahead. These could only be addressed and solved by two people, Krish and myself. I hoped that I would be able to convey Krish's and my deep concerns to the committee in a reassuring manner. This was my personal directive as I prepared for the committee's first meeting in seven weeks' time.

On May 27, 1980 the following telex was received from Madras: "Recd yr tlx many thanks. I am grateful for your efforts in getting approval from Rotary International. Started procedure for approvals from Delhi and hold harmless agreement. Shall advise later. Chitale."

Chairman Paul received formal approval of the project in a letter from John Stucky on June 19. John Stucky in his wisdom forwarded me a copy of this letter. The important information read as follows:

> The board agrees that US $405,100 be approved for the development and implementation of a program for red measles immunization in India, subject to the following conditions:
>
> [a] US $303,825.00 [three-quarters of the total budget of $405,100] be funded by the Canadian International Development Agency (CIDA);
> [b] Assurance will be given of involvement of Rotarian volunteers from several countries, as well as local Rotarians;
> [c] The participating Rotarian volunteers will develop a plan for the evaluation of immediate effects and long-term impact of the red measles immunization campaign.

On June 10 the Chairman of Trustees of The Rotary Foundation signed approval of the grant. The release of the funds has not been requested, since Rotary has not yet received the 'hold harmless' agreement from India. We have sent another telex to S.L. Chitale in Madras requesting that this be sent as soon as possible. In addition to the conditions contained in the board's decision, several additional administrative matters should be clarified for the record. District 707 will:

> [a] assume major administrative and management responsibility for the project through an appointed project management committee;

- Summer 1980 -

[b] formally notify the R.I. 3H program of results of district assembly action on the project and of management committee members;
[c] select volunteers for project (of which approximately 50 percent will be from non-USCB countries), from a volunteer list supplied by R.I.;
[d] establish an account into which CIDA and R.I. funds can be deposited and notify R.I. of procedure and timetable for deposit of funds;
[e] provide a periodic accounting of program expenditures and a project report to the 3H committee and to CIDA as required;
[f] arrange procurement of vaccines and of their transportation to destination point, and
[g] clarify relationships with District 320 (CIDA application draft prepared at R.I. listed present and incoming district governors of 320 as persons responsible in country);
[h] obtain written confirmation of responsible person in India (the stronger support at district level declared through district administrative action and measurable through the district's past and future activities, the more likely the achievement of the basic objectives of the 3H program); and
[i] send R.I. 3H program office a copy of the revised CIDA application.

The Rotary International 3H program staff will:

[a] assist the management committee in the coordination of the project;
[b] arrange for the deposit of approved funds when 'hold harmless' agreement is received from India;

and

[c] refer Rotary volunteers to be utilized in the project and secure signed volunteer agreement forms for those suggested by the 707 management committee.

Signed, John Stucky, Manager, Health, Hunger, and Humanity Program.

The two major requirements in order to proceed were: 1) signed hold harmless agreements from the states of Tamil Nadu and Kerala, and 2) agreement by Air India to transport the vaccine free of charge from New York to Madras. I challenged Krish to secure these two items before our August 16th meeting. However, this was not to be.

Following our meeting I wrote to Krish:

> Merck, Sharpe and Dohme, the manufacturer of the vaccine, has informed me that each shipment of 500,000 doses of Attenuvax [red measles vaccine] will contain 47 cartons, with a total weight of 5600 pounds, and will occupy 383 cubic feet.
>
> Eva and I will leave for India at our own expense on September the 23rd. We plan on arriving in New Delhi on October the 3rd and will be staying at the Maurya Sheraton in New Delhi. Please line up appropriate officials to see. Hopefully the first shipment of vaccine will arrive during my stay in Madras.

Merck, Sharpe and Dohme had earlier confirmed their anticipated shipment of vaccine as follows:

October 1980   500,000 doses
March 1981   500,000 doses

· Summer 1980 ·

September 1981   1 million doses
March 1982   1 million doses
September 1982   500,000 doses

The matter of the "hold harmless" agreement continued to plague me. The sum of my expectations rose on September 4, 1980, when Krish telexed: "This morning Tamil Nadu government agreed to sign hold harmless agreement. Will receive agreement on Monday. Krish."

The following week I was again in the doldrums when the following telex arrived:

> Hope you have received my previous telexes, anticipate some problem with civil aviation authorities. Could you urgently contact Rtn. Dr. Rostogi or Mr. Soni of Indian consulate Montreal and rush information regarding precedent for free transportation of medicine to India as gift. You may try R.I. if such information is available with them. Krish.

I replied to him on September 17 by telex:

> Dr. Rostogi and Mr. Soni report governor of state of Tamil Nadu must personally call federal minister of health, New Delhi, requesting him to sanction civil aviation lift free of charge gift 3 1/2 million doses red measles vaccine worth approx. 4 million US dollars New York-Bombay-Madras in 6 shipments. First shipment approx. Oct. 24/80. Last year's small shipment paid by manufacturer, precedent Red Cross supplies of lesser value have been transported free. Signed, Ken Hobbs.

Echoes of August '79 were reverberating. I received the following telex on September 19, four days before our proposed departure for

India: "Suggest you postpone your 23rd departure, until you receive advice from us. Pls send your tour programme. Signed, Krish Chitale."

Fortunately I was now part South Indian, and I realized that all would work out. As Krish had told me many times before, "This is India, Ken. One has to have a great deal of commitment and patience. If you have, all will be well."

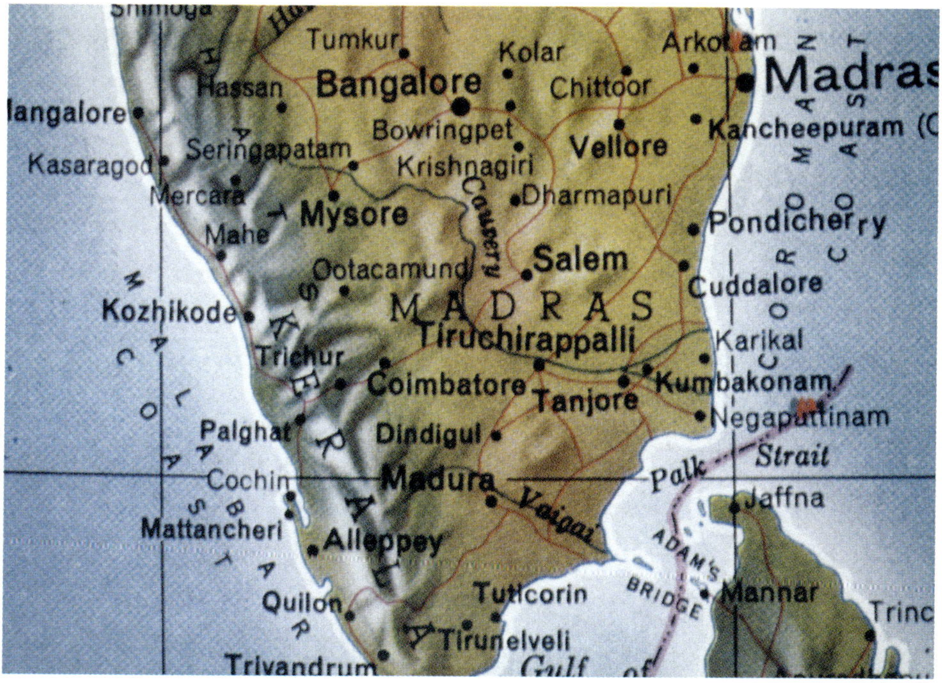

Map of the states of Tamil Nadu and Kearala, South India.

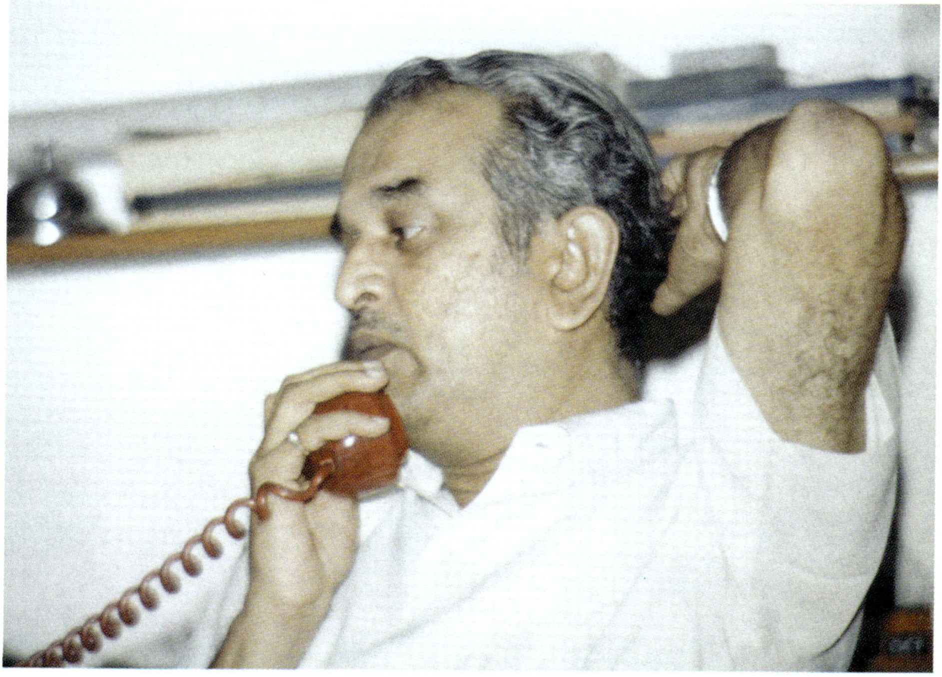

Rotarian Krish Chitale—"Mr. Measles"—the motivator of the massive immunization project in South India.

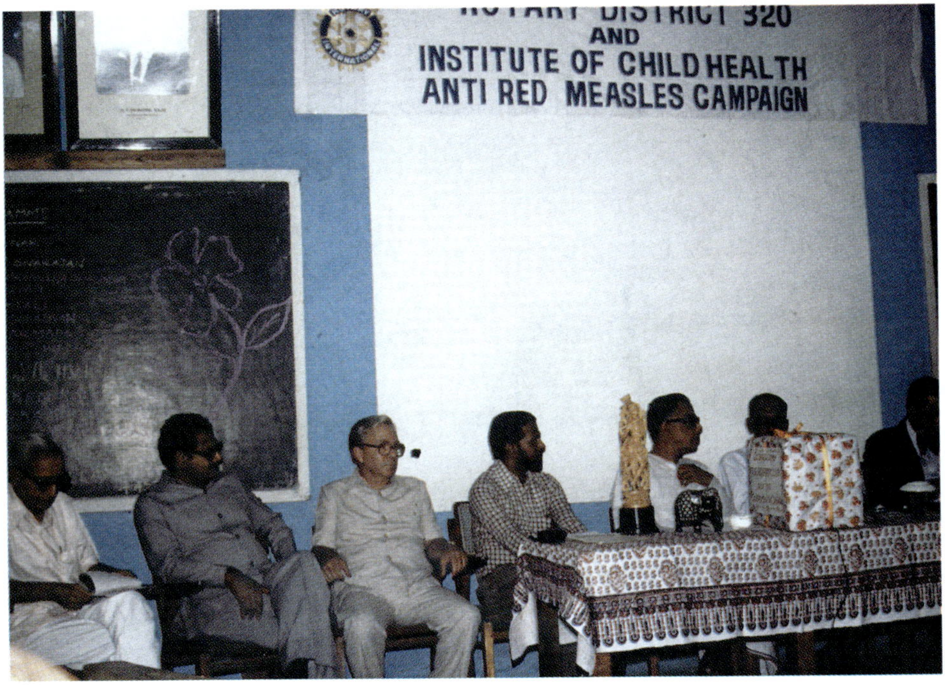

Indian Medical Association's symposium on measles, September 22, 1979.

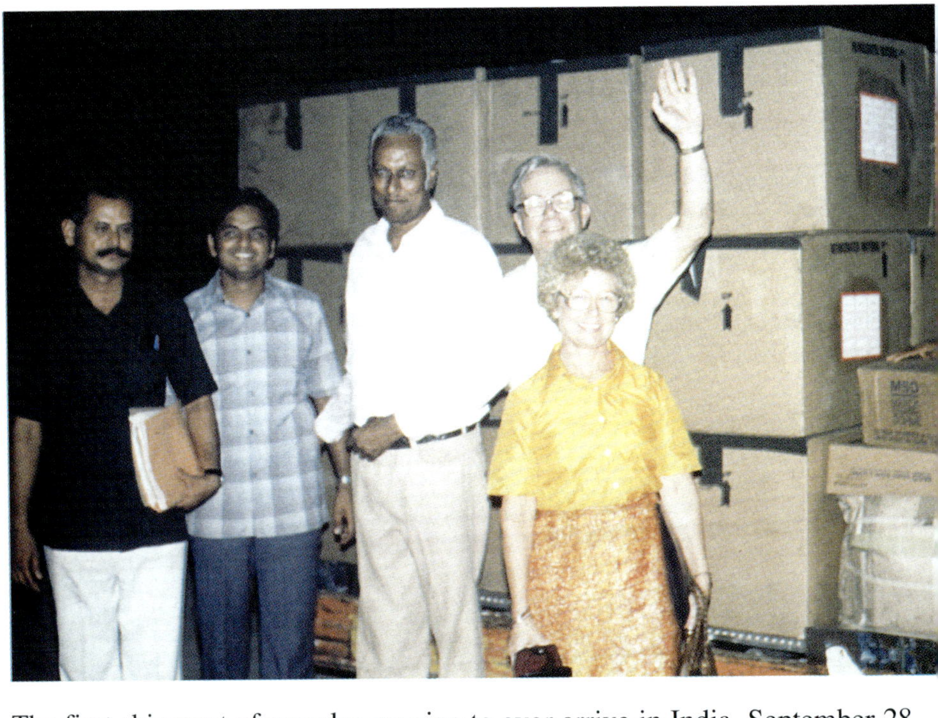

The first shipment of measles vaccine to ever arrive in India, September 28, 1979.

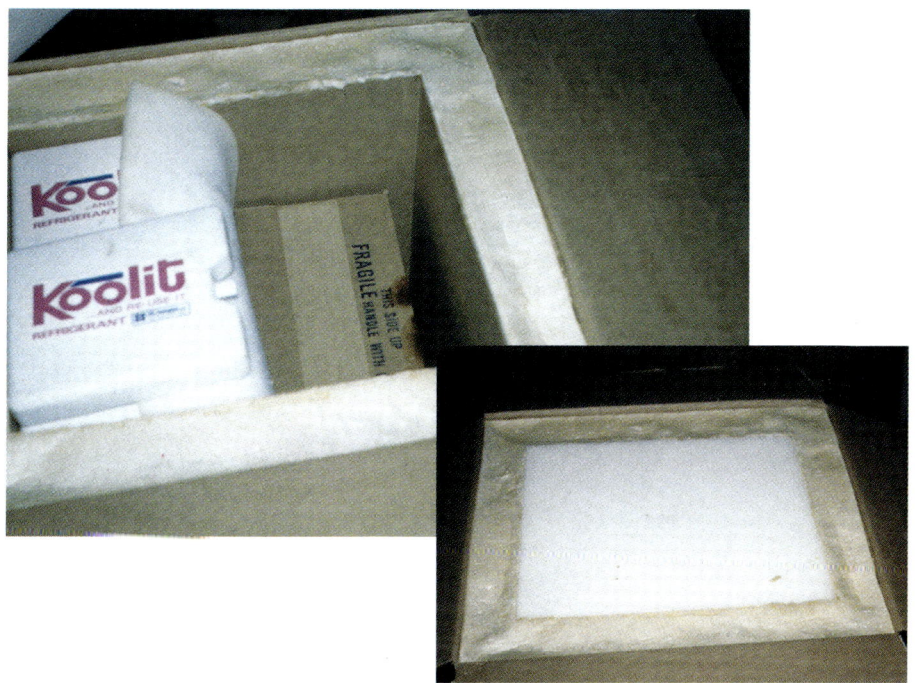

Packaging of measles vaccine for transport from New York to Madras, in order for the vaccine to be kept frozen.

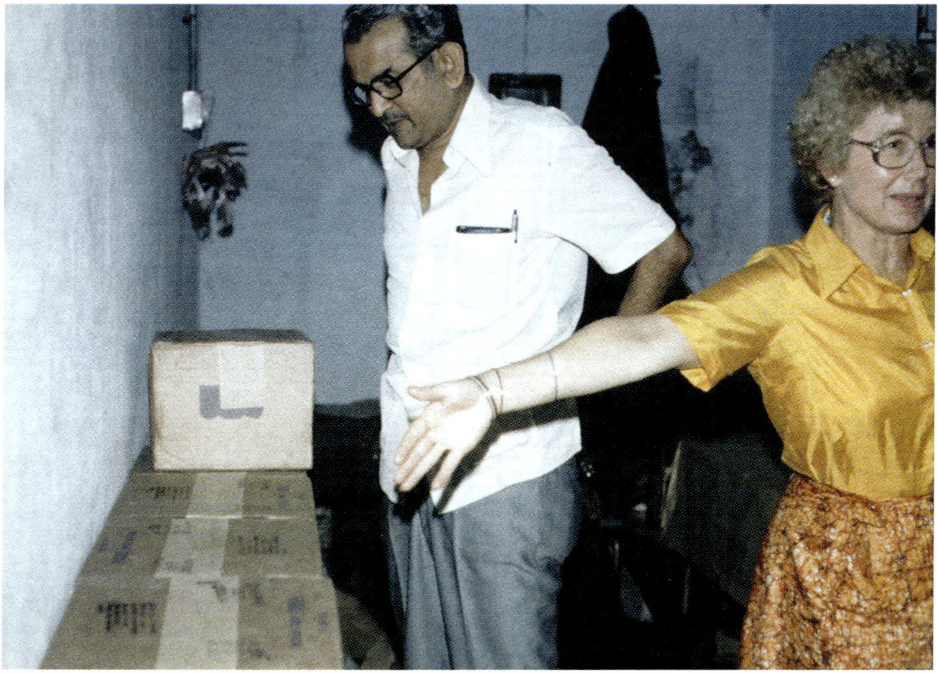

Unpacking the vaccine on September 29, 1979, at Spencer's Store in Madras.

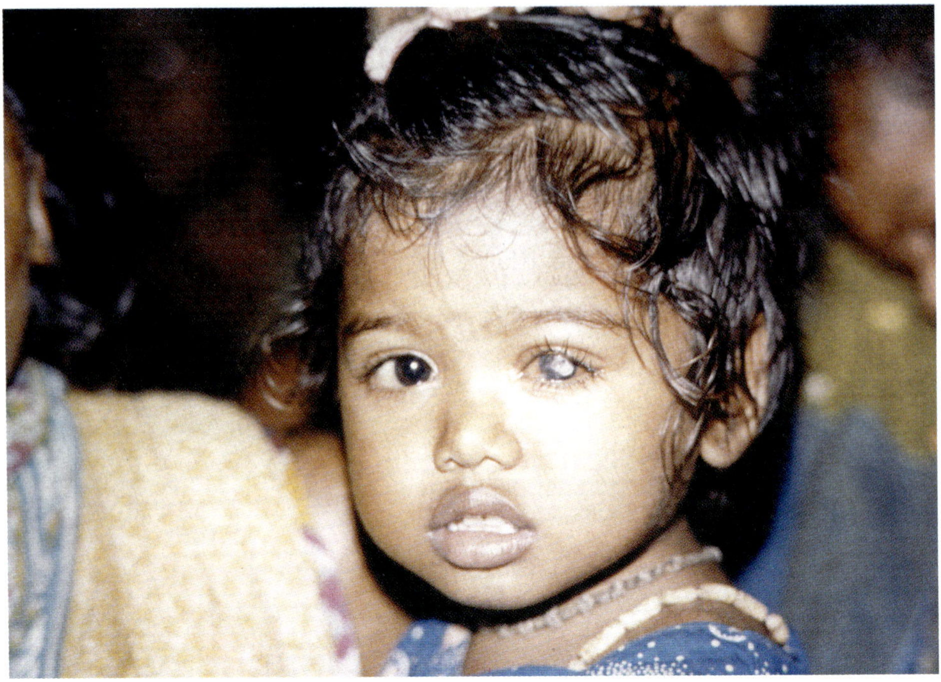

A patient of Dr. Vankataswami in Madurai, South India, who had developed a cataract as a sequelae from measles.

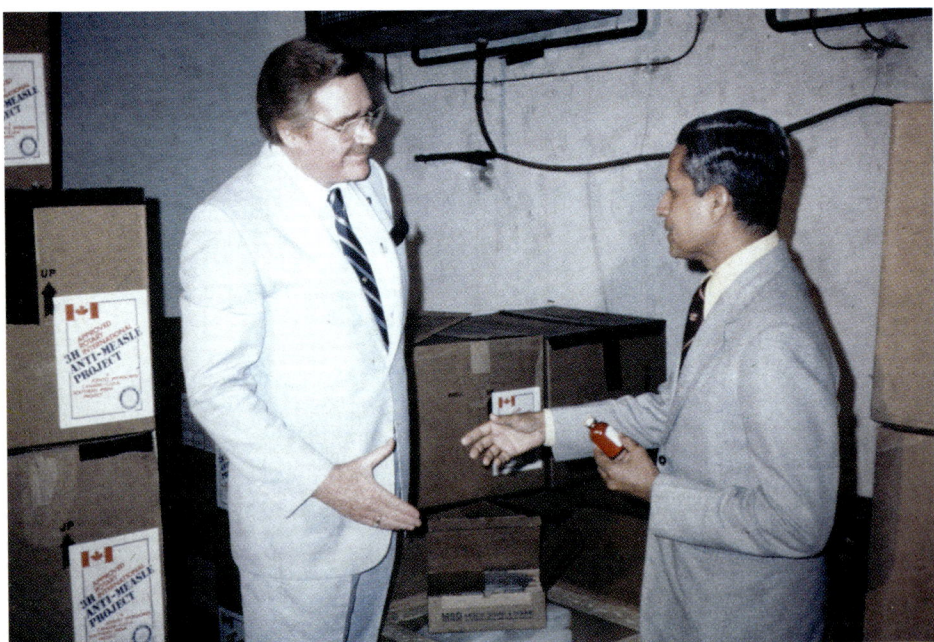

Governor Fran Smith of Scarborough, Ontario, the first committee member to volunteer, inspects the recently arrived vaccine with a Ministry of Health official in the standby refrigeration unit.

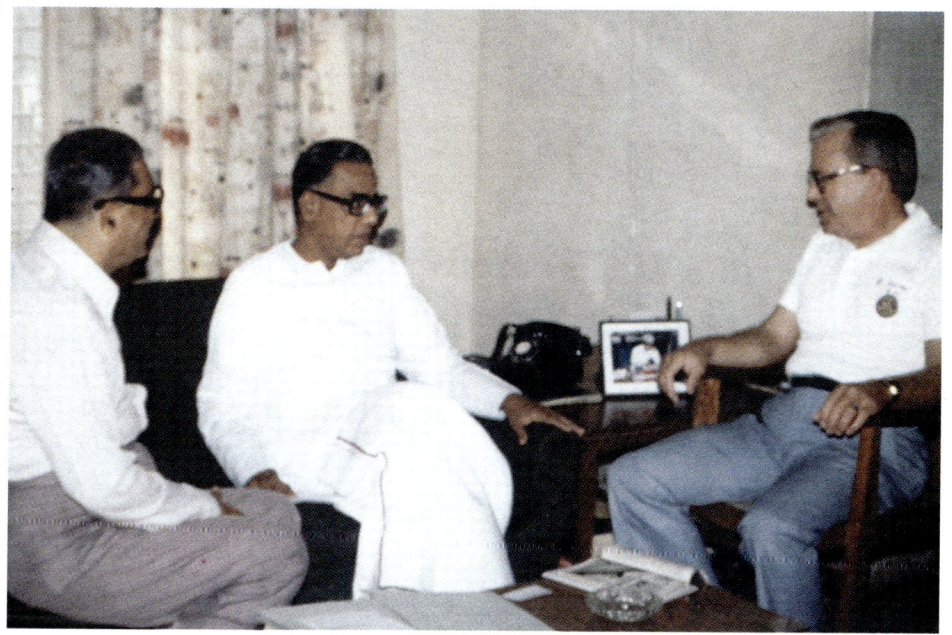

Rotarians Dr. Pillay and Dr. Ken Hobbs discuss the infrastructure needed for the massive immunization project with Dr. Hande, Minister of Health, February 1982.

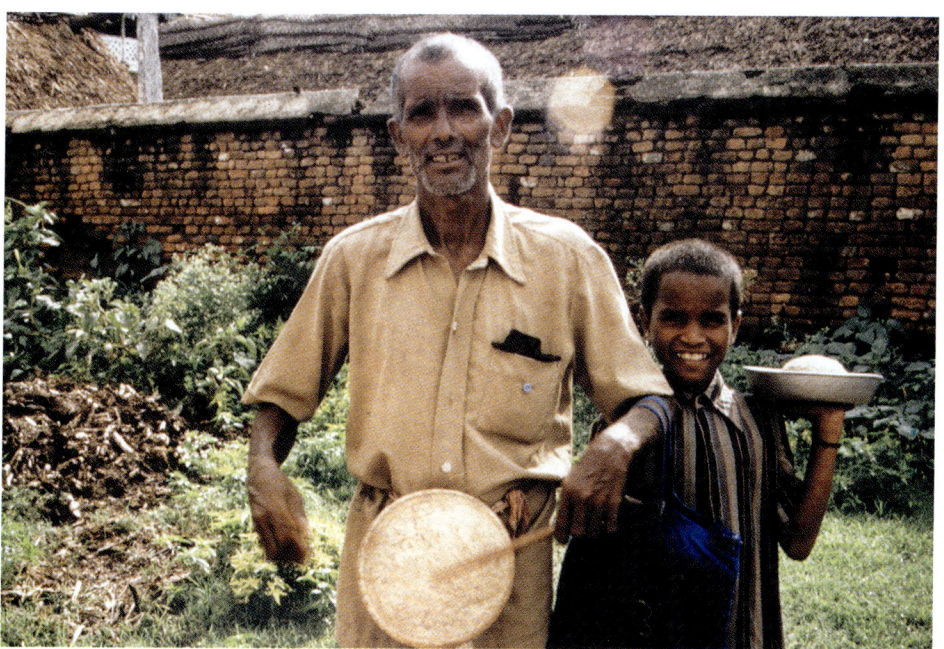

Town crier beating the drum for mothers to bring their children to the measles immunization camp.

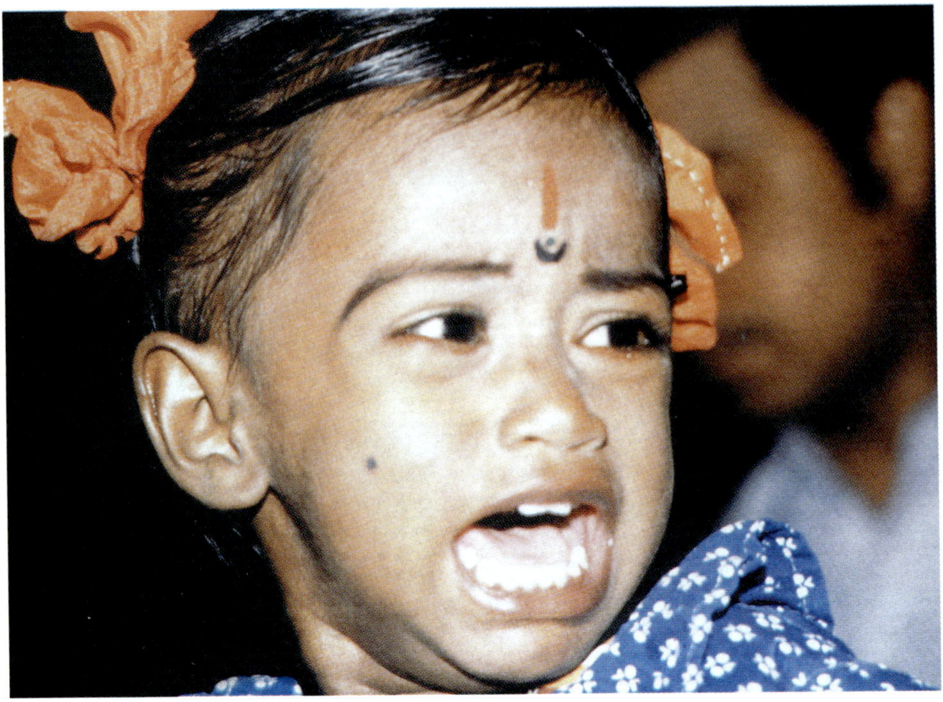

It hurts!

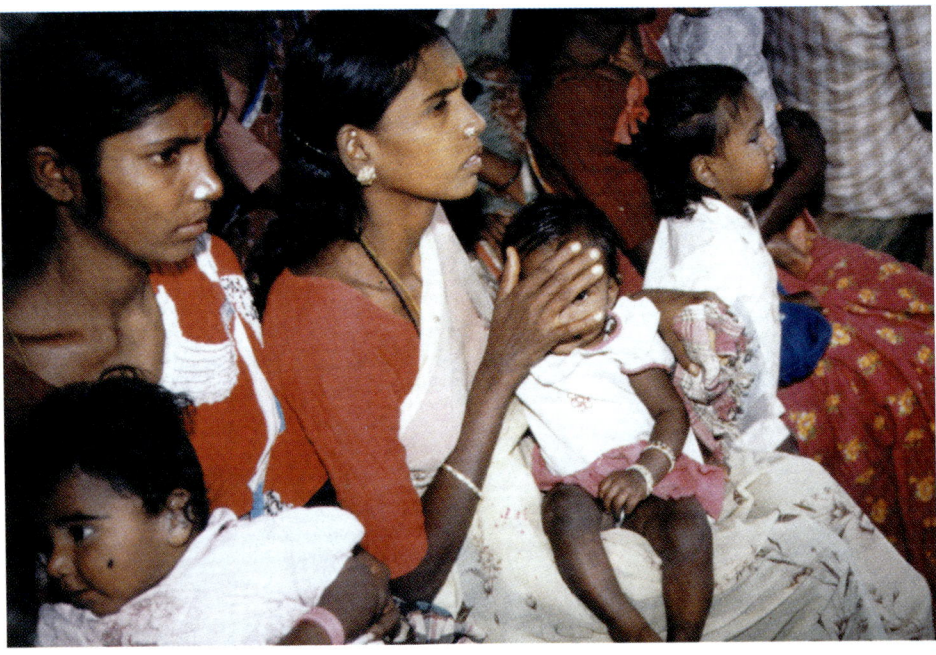

Mothers patiently waiting at an immunization camp.

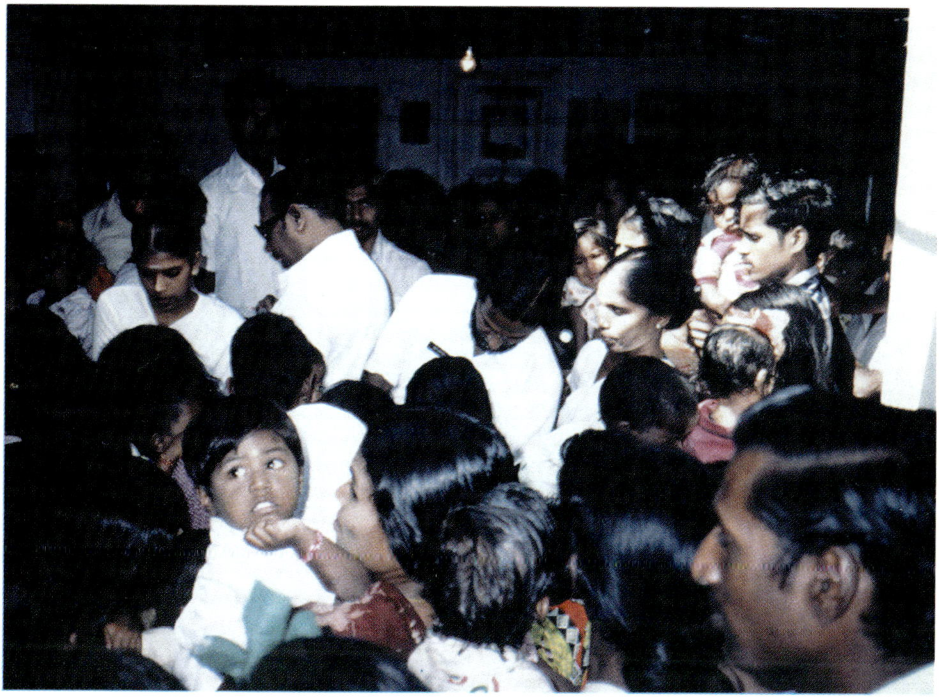

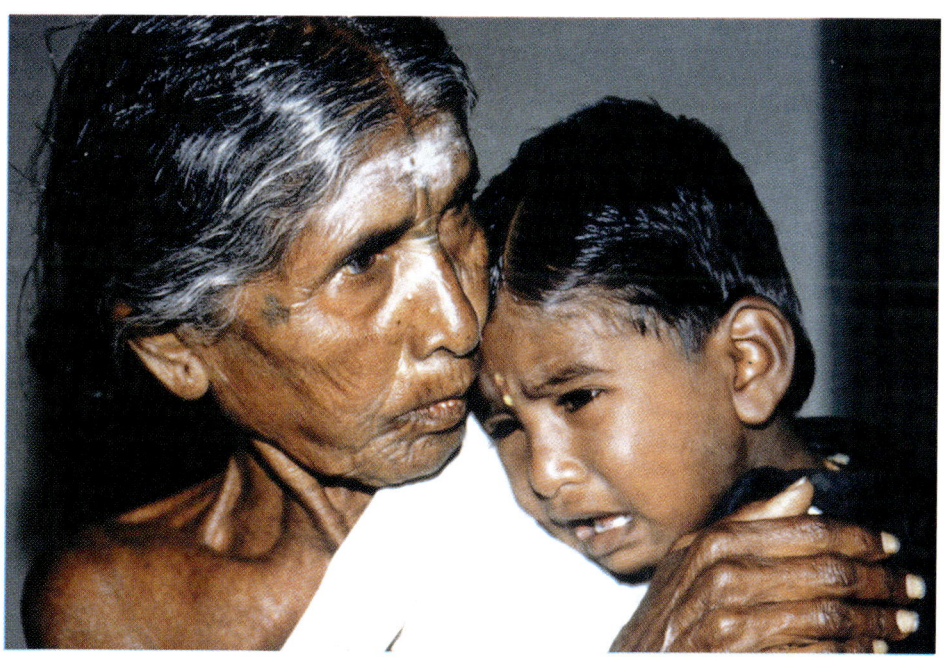

A typical measles immunization camp.

Grandmother thanks Rotary for protecting her grandson from the ravages of measles.

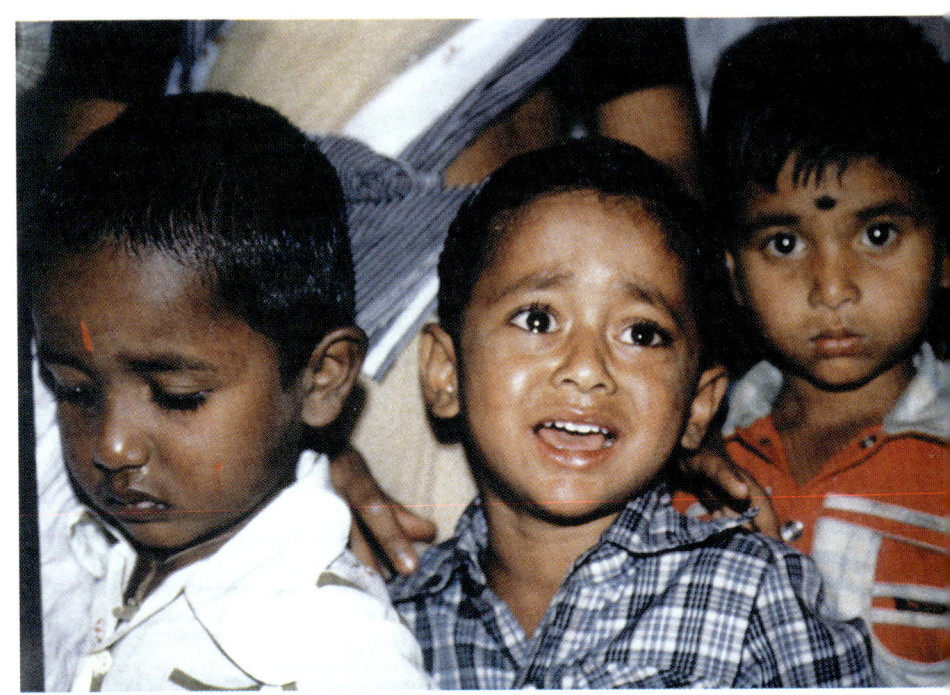

Thank you!

Chapter 17

My reply to Krish's telex of September 19 was concise and definite. It read:

> Too much at stake for India to cancel or postpone my Sept. 23 departure. Hold harmless must go to Stucky at Rotary International immediately or project is dead. Will help on my arrival. Street value of vaccine in Canada is 14 million USA dollars. Sept. 23-29 Germany, Sept. 30 Intercontinental Hotel Frankfurt Airport. Oct. 1-3 Intercontinental Hotel Karachi. Oct. 3-6 Maurya Hotel New Delhi. Keep the faith and working at the project. Signed, Ken Hobbs.

When I awoke on the morning of October 1 in my Frankfurt hotel room, I discovered a message from Krish under my door. "Hold harmless agreements signed and sent to John Stucky in Evanston. Will phone you morning of your arrival in New Delhi."

My faith in Krish's ability was once again confirmed. We arrived in New Delhi at three in the morning on Saturday, October 4. It seemed as if I had just fallen asleep when the phone rang. It was 6:30 a.m. The loud, cheery voice said: "Wake up! You're not on holiday. The driver will pick you up at nine. I have a full day lined up for you. First he will take you sightseeing around New Delhi. Then a friend of mine will pick you up at the hotel on Sunday morning and spend the day with you and

Eva. You will have supper at his home. Enjoy yourselves! I will call with instructions for your itinerary on Monday morning." Before I could truly comprehend what he had said, Krish hung up.

I hadn't realized that you had a maximum of only three minutes for some long distance telephone calls, but this was brought home to me over the next couple of days when I attempted to call Krish in Madras. There are three types of calls: emergency calls, priority calls, and ordinary calls. And you can't just dial. You have to book the call, stating what kind you want; the operator will then give you a precise time when the call may be placed. Not knowing what the consequences would be, I booked an ordinary call. This type of call lasts only for a maximum of three minutes. When the allotted time is over the operator will terminate your call with no warning.

The other two types of calls can last a maximum of six minutes. On my previous visit I had not used the telephone. This was my first experience of the operator's authoritative ways.

The weekend was very pleasant. Eva and I spent a great deal of time at Mahatma Gandhi's home and museum. They had a wealth of film clips on his life. They had also marked his last steps in his garden, just before he was assassinated.

That evening I had a long and fascinating talk with our guide, Krish's friend, about Gandhi. He was very knowledgeable about the Mahatma, who was familiarly known as Baptu. In his opinion, Gandhi should have created an irrigation canal from the Himalayas in the north to Trivandrum in the south. This could have been done right after Independence when there was a scarcity of work and wages were very low. This idea has always stuck in my mind as an excellent one, especially in view of the absence of any sort of water conservation projects, and the scarcity of an adequate water supply in India today.

On Monday at 6:30 a.m., the phone rang again. "Ken. Krish here. I hope you have enjoyed your holiday. Today is a work day. The driver will be at the hotel sharp at 9:00 a.m. Don't keep him waiting! Your itinerary

New Dehli, September 1980

today begins with a visit to the Canadian embassy. You have an appointment with Mr. Murray Esselmont at 9:30. He is the development officer at the Canadian high commissioner's office. Following this appointment, the driver will take you to visit Dr. Tong, the director of the Volunteer Health Association for India. Mr. Murray Esselment has set up this interview for you and Eva.

"Next, I have scheduled a visit with Mr. Harry Lucker, the UNICEF director for India. In the afternoon, just before lunch, you will visit Dr. Rajit Sen, deputy director of health services for India."

The next thing I heard was a loud knock on the door. I turned over and noticed that the time was 9:00 a.m. As I went to the door I could hear a voice saying, "Your driver is here, sir. I will wait downstairs for you." We were downstairs as quickly as possible—within half an hour. The driver approached us. He was a Sikh, about thirty years of age, and very pleasant. He spoke impeccable English.

When we arrived at the Canadian embassy, the receptionist escorted us to the office of Mr. Esselmont, the counselor for development in the embassy. He apologized to us for the absence of Mr. Fernandez, the NGO development officer for CIDA, who was in South India on business. Our discussions with Mr. Esselmont were very rewarding. He was fully informed about our initial project for red measles immunization. We talked at great length regarding the difficulties I had experienced with the Indian government last year, both at the state and federal levels. He remarked that as I was now accustomed to Indian ways, all should proceed with less difficulty this year. He did not in so many words commit the Canadian government to providing funding, but he expressed his own warm approval of our new, enlarged 3.5-million-dose 3H Rotary project, and indicated that he felt that CIDA would certainly become a partner in this humanitarian project. In short, he left us in little doubt that all would soon be approved; in parting, he wished us good luck.

Next, our driver delivered us to the office of Dr. Tong, the director of the Volunteer Health Association of India. He, too, was fully cognizant of the red measles project of the previous year. He voiced his gratitude that an organization such as Rotary International had embarked on a mission of red measles immunization, and he emphasized that the necessity of such a program could not be overstated. He was very impressed with the initial organization and in particular the "cold chain" (the term refers to the methodology that we had employed, utilizing 100 percent refrigeration, with adequate backup electrical power via automatic generator). He thanked us for all of our interest in the children of South India.

Mr. Harry Lucker was our next appointment. He was the director of UNICEF in India. Our first impression, on entering his very luxurious office, was that he appeared aloof and cool. Mr. Lucker seemed to be looking at us suspiciously, and taking our measure.

At the outset of our conversation I tried to convey to him that Rotary International was not attempting to take over the federal ministry of health or UNICEF's role in providing health care for the children of India; our only aim was to reinforce the work of the federal government and UNICEF, as it related to red measles immunization.

Mr. Lucker appeared unconvinced. Striking a rather arrogant attitude, he stated, "Dr. Hobbs, you are using the wrong strain of vaccine."

Here it was again. The war between the Swartz and Edmonston strain was not over yet. I assured him that the information he had about Attenuvax, the vaccine we had used in South India in 1979, was inaccurate. "I would suggest, sir," I said politely, " that you look up in your files the type of vaccine used in UNICEF's limited survey of the efficacy of red measles vaccine in India."

As he pawed through his disorganized files, I sat in perplexity, wondering what he on earth he would find. He stopped at one particular page for a long time. I was able to peer over his desk and read upside down the words "Merck, Sharpe and Dohme."

"I believe you will find, sir, that you did use the Attenuvax strain in your limited survey," I continued, "though I hardly feel that 500 doses of vaccine constitutes a sufficient survey."

He looked over his glasses at me, grudgingly, and continued to read a

· New Dehli, September 1980 ·

report from his files, but as he read a look of interest appeared on his face, and he seemed to realize that he had made a mistake.

We continued our conversation, and by the end of the meeting he had become quite warm and sincere. We discussed how many doses would constitute the basis of a reasonable survey for the federal ministry of health. He explained that it was mandatory that a conclusive survey be done before any approval of a massive immunization program against red measles in all of India could be given. I now felt that we were indeed in the driver's seat. However, I realized that there would be more roadblocks put in my way either by Mr. Lucker or some other government bureaucrat.

"Perhaps a minimum of 10,000 doses per shipment would be adequate," I suggested.

"Perhaps," was his reply.

I felt that this gift would fall within the parameters we had originally set out in our application to CIDA. We had emphatically stated that in the long term, India would have to produce or import its own vaccine. I personally felt that this gift of 10,000 doses per shipment, which would amount to 60,000 doses over the entire project, was justified. On our departure he assured me that the UNICEF representative in Madras would aid the Rotarians in the project.

After lunch we visited with Dr. Rajit Sen, the deputy director of health services. He had granted the import license for the vaccine last year and was also responsible for waiving the import duties. He had been surprised and extremely pleased, he told us, by the success of the 1979 project in District 320. The card control system that Krish had used had also impressed Dr. Sen. He voiced the hope that the Rotarians might also, in the future, include the department of health's DPT (diphtheria, pertussis [whooping cough], and tetanus) and BCG (tuberculosis) vaccines. I promised that I would attempt to accommodate his request. Our interview ended on a very congenial note. He thanked me sincerely and eloquently for Rotary's concern for the health of India's children.

Back at the hotel, we were greeted with a message: a gracious invitation to join Mr. Esselmont, of the Canadian embassy, and his wife for dinner that evening. We accepted this invitation with pleasure. The evening was most enjoyable, as the Esselmonts had other Canadian guests.

Tuesday morning brought the same routine. The phone rang at 6:30 a.m., and Krish loudly gave me my instructions. The driver would arrive at nine o'clock sharp. Today we were to visit Dr. Pierre Ziegler, regional director of the expanded program of immunization administered by WHO. Dr. Ziegler was most emphatic in his enthusiasm for Rotary's involvement in the attempted eradication of red measles, which he said had been overlooked and ignored both in India and throughout the Far East for too long. He expressed his respect and appreciation for Dr. Jacob John's skills, and praised his exemplary professional dedication. He unequivocally stated that with Dr. Jacob John involved, the project would be a success.

Dr. Ziegler also expressed his appreciation for the effort and dedication that had gone into maintaining the "cold chain" in the pilot project. He further stated, categorically, that our work would set the standard for any future red measles eradication programs, not only in India, but in Africa and Southeast Asia as well.

Our last interview before leaving in early evening for Madras was perhaps the most significant. This was with Mr. Sharma, the minister of civil aviation and tourism. We had a favor to ask of him. Rotary International had stipulated that the vaccine must be transported free by Air India from New York to Madras. The precedent for free shipment of vaccine had been set in 1979 when a shipment of tetanus toxoid, donated by Connaught Labs in Toronto, had been shipped free of charge by Canadian Pacific Airlines from Toronto to Manila in the Philippines. I was not aware of another mandate for free transport of vaccines since.

I felt strained as we walked into the minister's office. He had kept us waiting outside for some forty-five minutes. His secretary informed us that he was busy discussing small aircraft purchases with a Canadian manufacturer.

New Dehli, September 1980

Eva and I were not alone for this encounter: accompanying us was a gentleman who was well versed in the ways of Indian government officials. Our companion was what you would call in our political circles a lobbyist: he knew how to play the game. And it was indeed a game. Over the past year I had learned just how far governmental interference and, at times, stupidity could go. Our assistant had been chosen by Kumar and endorsed by Krish. Kumar required the most knowledgeable, sophisticated and wisest of support staff when he was attempting to get approvals in his chemical and drug manufacturing business.

In the minister's inner sanctum, a pair of harried eyes were lifted to us, from a desk that had voluminous amounts of paper scattered on it.

"I am in a very great hurry. Please be brief. What can I do for you?"

I started to spell out why we were there and what I hoped he could do. I referred to the shipment of last September, which had not been shipped free of charge. I stressed the need for this vaccine, and its great value: it was worth $14 million (US). I explained why it was needed and the number of children's lives it would save. He thanked me, and turned away. It seemed that the interview was over. We stood up and began to say our good-byes.

However, at the door, I asked the gentleman who accompanied us to return quickly and ask the minister whether he would approve the shipments of vaccine from New York to Madras.

Eva and I waited while the professional lobbyist did his work. On his return he exclaimed, "He will sign the order for free transport, and will forward it to Mr. Chitale tomorrow."

What the minister did not know was that Krish had arranged for Eva and me to meet with Prime Minister Indira Gandhi the next morning. If Mr. Sharma had not consented to free transportation of the vaccine by Air India, we would have gone over his head, and asked her.

Chapter 18

Before leaving the Maurya Hotel for Madras, I received a telex from Bill Nurse in Whitby: "CIDA approved and signed. Awaiting reply from Stucky. If agreement is in his hands it will be okay to go ahead with shipping arrangements."

In Madras we were met with the usual pomp and ceremony at the airport: garlanding, handshakes, embraces from Krish, his wife, and our other friends. The prodigal son couldn't have had a finer reception on his return home. Adula, Krish's driver, asked for our luggage slips, picked up our suitcases and loaded them in the car. Adula is a sweet, gracious man, whom we had got to know well on our previous trip. Krish's father had employed him after the death of Krish's mother, thirty-eight years ago, as a companion for Krish, and he is still a member of the household. He acts as a chauffeur and general servant, and he will likely continue to do so for as long as he lives.

On arriving home, Krish handed me the current information on the project. A telex from John Stucky:

> Tamil Nadu agreement okay. Measles program approved by Rotary International. Kerala agreement alterations unacceptable. Do not send any measles vaccine to Kerala until Rotary's hold harmless agreement is signed and approved by Rotary International. Could you use possible donation of 250,000 doses of tetanus toxoid in 5 ml vials expiring in February 1981? If yes telex urgent

shipping instructions, address and quantity. Signed, John Stucky."

And a second telex from Bill Nurse:

"McKelvey advises Merck Sharpe and Dohme will not have serum available until end of January.

Krish decided that we should now relax and enjoy our hospitality hour and worry about measles in the morning. The next three weeks would pass very quickly. Eva and I were kept busy with meetings in Madras and trips elsewhere: to Vellore; to Coimbatore to visit District Governor G. Vadaraj and his wife Shree; a district governor's visit to Ooty; and visits to Madurai, Trichur, Cochin, and Trivandrum. After these visits I could truly say that we had visited the main centers of South India in the states of Kerala and Tamil Nadu.

Two days after our arrival Krish and I had a meeting with Dr. Jacob John and three other Rotarians from the Vellore Rotary Club. We concluded that the first shipment should arrive in Madras between January 19 and 22, 1981. This would coincide with the district conference which was to be held in Coimbatore four days later. The upcoming plans for the seminar that was scheduled for Trichur were discussed at length. Dr. Nair of Trichur would be instrumental in organizing this seminar. Dr C.R. Pillay of Madras, who was chairman of the District 320 committee, would act as chairman of the seminar.

Dr. Jacob John invited me to Vellore to witness a red measles camp; Eva and I accepted this invitation with a deep sense of gratitude. We had been trying for the past sixteen months to bring about the creation of the vaccination program. Now, for the first time, we would be able to witness the reality of what we had created.

Government officials, of course, still caused us delay and frustration at every turn. For the first time I met Dr. B. Padmanabhan, the assistant director of health services of Tamil Nadu. He was most enthusiastic concerning our expanded program, and he was also in full agreement with

Dr. Jacob John's assessment regarding the destructiveness of red measles in South India. Also in attendance at this meeting was Dr. Thirughansambandan, whom I had met last year when he was the deputy director of the Institute of Child Health. He was now responsible for undertaking a survey for the ministry of health, concerning measles. Much to my surprise he openly suggested that Rotary should and could contribute financially to this survey. He suggested that we should contribute 20,000 rupees ($3,000). I was shocked at his quick turnaround from a year ago, when he had openly opposed our initial 68,000-dose project. Now he was asking us for funds to do a red measles survey! I suggested that he write me a letter asking for Rotary's financial help. I assured him that I personally would follow up on his request. Two days later I received his written request. This, I believe, was the first time that a government official in South India had ever requested financial help from Rotary International in writing.

Our flight to Coimbatore on the early morning of October 12, 1980, was delightful. We first flew to Bangalore, where we were met by a group of local Rotarians, then after a brief stop departed for Coimbatore.

On arrival in Coimbatore we were greeted by Governor G.V. and his wife Shree, whom we had met when they visited us in Whitby the previous June, after the Chicago International Rotary Convention. The usual Indian traditions of garlanding and the giving of mementos followed. In customary fashion the day's activities were outlined by one of G.V.'s aides. We would be going to G.V. and Shree's home for a brief stop, then proceeding by car to Ooty, which was in the mountains at the 7500-foot level—a two-and-a-half-hour car ride, with twenty-six hairpin turns.

Their home reflected their station in life. G.V. was a very successful industrialist and the head of a large family-run educational charity, which had been started by his grandfather, father and three uncles some fifty years before. I could not know then that their home would be our home whenever we visited Coimbatore over the following fifteen years. Governor G.V., like Krish Chitale, was very warm and unassuming. He had the ability to make you feel at home, as though you were a part of the family who had just arrived after a lengthy absence.

Our car journey up the mountain was tedious. Every one of the sharp hairpin turns was marked and numbered. The driver and the Mercedes made the trip bearable. Shree kept telling me that I was making a mistake in not accepting one of G.V.'s sweaters, but I kept insisting I was a true Canadian and never ever complained about cold weather. I was assuming that since the temperature in Madras had been 95 degrees Fahrenheit, with 95 percent humidity, anything cooler would be a welcome experience. Indians, I thought, didn't know what real cold was. Little did I know what was in store for me.

On our arrival in Ooty we were met by a large contingent of Rotarians. G.V. told me during our long trip that I would be inaugurating a housing project which had been funded by Districts 701, 704 and 707. The settlements had been devastated by a cyclone and landslide that went through the area in 1978. Eighteen housing units had been reconstructed by Rotary, with CIDA (Canadian International Development Agency) funding, for eighteen senior Ooty residents. As I stood in the open, under a gray sky, with the cold wind blowing, I was sharply reminded of Shree's offer of one of G.V.'s sweaters. Why, I wondered now, had I been such a fool as to refuse?

That evening at the YMCA, during G.V.'s governor's address, I eyed the brightly burning fire in the old fireplace. The crackling of the logs was indeed a welcome sound. I edged as close as I could, wondering if perhaps I should indeed jump in and get warm. Never in my life had I been colder.

On this brief visit to Coimbatore I had the privilege of visiting Bhavani, a community some seventy-five miles south of Coimbatore. It was like walking centuries back into Indian history. I was greeted by the warmest people I have ever met. A handmade rug was presented to Eva and me, personally inscribed, which still hangs on our wall at home.

We visited a small reclaimed village. As in Ooty, I was met by the head official of the village, who bent down to kiss my feet. This struck me as being embarrassingly subservient. I immediately stepped back and knelt to kiss his feet, which were bare, worn, bruised and soil-stained. He shook his head, saying, "No, no, no." We embraced and walked towards the center of the village hand in hand. I mention this incident to show how deeply grateful these poor villagers are for what Rotary has done for them. It re-emphasized to me the importance and respect our organization called Rotary has earned. At that moment I rededicated myself to the ideals expressed in our mottoes: "Service above Self" and "He profits most who serves best."

The morning after our return to Madras I was introduced to the most powerful and respected industrialist in all of South India. Mr. J.K. Devarju is better know as JKD. Krish was designing a very large industrial building for him in the Coimbatore area. As I entered his Madras home and office, we were greeted by a young houseboy, who ushered us into the reception area. Shortly thereafter a large, portly, smiling individual in his early seventies, dressed in a cotton *dhoti*, entered the room. Krish rose and introduced me to him. His handshake was warm and forceful.

"Please, sit down," he urged us, and we did so. Krish began to give JKD an update on the building plans. JKD rang his side bell, and another fine young, barefoot servant entered the room.

"What will you have to drink, Dr. Hobbs?"

"Nothing, thank you," I replied.

"Oh, but you must have something," JKD protested. "It is now 11:15 in the morning. We South Indians prefer gin before noon." With this he gave instructions to the servant, who disappeared for a few minutes. When he reappeared he was carrying two crystal glasses with a slice of lime in each.

"Cheers, Dr. Hobbs." He and Krish resumed their conversation without dropping a verb.

I forced myself to sip the (very strong) gin and tonic that had been placed in my hand, but before I was finished it, I was again confronted with an invitation from the hospitable elderly gentleman.

"Another gin, Dr. Hobbs?"

"No, I'm fine, perfectly fine."

"But I was not asking about your state of health!" He smiled broadly, and went on, "Are you a friend, Dr. Hobbs?"

"Yes, sir," I answered.

"Then you must know that I never offer a second drink to anyone who is not a friend!" With that, he summoned the servant, who brought me another gin and tonic. After they were finished discussing their business the conversation turned to why I was in South India. Krish explained that this was my second visit and that I had paid my own way. Rotary, he told JKD, was now embarking on an expanded 3.5-million-dose red measles immunization project.

It came up in conversation that I was a member of the Masonic Order. On hearing that, our host very cordially asked, "When are you coming to Coimbatore?"

"In ten days " I replied.

JKD immediately turned, picked up the phone and called Bombay. After speaking briefly to someone in that city, he said to Krish, "It's all set. Dr. Hobbs has been cleared to speak at the lodge in Coimbatore in ten days' time. The grandmaster of India has just given his consent to this special meeting."

This was perhaps the first time in the modern history of Rotary International that a Rotarian had been invited by a Mason to speak in open Masonic lodge in order to ask its members for their assistance with a Rotary International project. And this would not be the last time our paths would cross. Several times over the next five years I would be granted the opportunity to visit and share fellowship with the dedicated industrialist known as JKD.

Our seminar in Trichur was an enormous success. Over 140 Rotarians, public health officials, government officials, pediatricians and other interested parties came from as far away as Madras and even from Trivandrum, the capital of the state of Kerala, which is situated almost at the tip of India. The enthusiasm exhibited by Dr. K.B. Nair, the organizer of this seminar and workshop, was refreshing, and his personal dedication to the project was enormous. His selfless commitment over the past eight months was an inspiration to all but a few of the Rotarians in the state of Kerala. However, I would meet a number of doubting Thomases over the next several days.

At the seminar, a short elderly social worker stood up, and had these thoughts to share with us. "You can all decide what the poor people will do. You can organize and regulate and legislate what they must do. But you must realize that they will not follow your instructions. However, they will follow my directions, because they know me and they trust me. They will follow what I will advise them to do. And I will advise them to immunize their children against red measles, because a doctor from Canada has paid his own way to bring this vaccine, and in order for him to make such a commitment to do this he must feel that it is good for our poor children of Kerala." With this statement she sat down to thunderous applause.

She later apologized to me for not speaking in proper English. She told me that she had not spoken English for the past twenty years, and also confided that she had never before in her life had the pleasure of addressing such a large assembly of government officials and medical doctors.

Our brief stay in Cochin was fruitless. It was soon quite obvious to all of us, Krish, Eva and myself, that what we had to say was falling on deaf ears. However, two younger Rotarians who had attended the workshop in Trichur promised me that they would push the project to the fullest extent of their power.

In Trivandrum I sampled several varieties of banana, raw and cooked, at a special breakfast reception hosted by the chief of pediatrics in Trivandrum. She warmly endorsed our program of red measles immunization. Following a very short meeting with the minister of health, I had the opportunity of meeting Dr. Sukkeranan, an ear, nose and throat (ENT) specialist, who is head of the pediatrics department at the medical college in Trivandrum. He was very enthusiastic and supportive of the program. He offered to send me a copy of a recent survey done at his medical school concerning red measles and deafness.

Shortly after our return to Madras I had the opportunity of meeting Dr. Hande, the minister of health for the state of Tamil Nadu. Our first meeting was short but pleasant. Our paths would cross several times over the next few years, and he would become not only a staunch supporter of the program but also, and more importantly, a very close personal friend. *[One of his important acts of assistance to the program will be recounted in Chapter 21.]*

We flew to Madurai to meet with Rotarian President Ramesh, a prominent young industrialist who was also a dedicated Rotarian. He had on several occasions been in touch with John Stucky in Evanston, wanting information about when and how the measles program was coming to District 321. Our discussions with Rotarian Ramesh were fruitful. He offered the use of his trucking facilities to transport the vaccine at any time, to or from any destination. He also suggested that I visit Dr. Vankataswami, a dedicated and prominent eye surgeon in Madurai.

Rotarian Ramesh had showed us movies of Dr. Vankataswami doing several complicated eye operations, so that the next day, on meeting Dr. Vankataswami, I was shocked to see that his hands were badly deformed from rheumatoid arthritis. However, his condition did not appear to hinder him in his delicate work.

Early in our conversations, Dr. Vankataswami reminded me that in order to have good health a child must have clean, potable water, clean air and red measles vaccine. We discussed in great detail the effect of red measles as a major cause of blindness in children under the age of five years. He stated that measles was the third cause of blindness in this age group. He showed me several youngsters now in his institution who had become blind due to red measles.

Our visit to Pondicherry, a former French colony situated some 120 miles south of Madras, was very interesting, but unfortunately I never reached first base as far as the local Rotarians were concerned. They seemed to have little interest in, or commitment to, the measles program.

In spite of our hectic schedule, I still had to deal with the possibility of a shipment of measles vaccine before we left Madras. I had received several telexes, the most important of which was dated October 14, 1980: "McKelvey has confirmed that 200,000 doses available for shipment the weeks of November 3. Advise if positive air freight data, prepaid or collect and package markings. Signed, Bill Nurse."

My reply was as follows: "Free shipment 1/2 million doses only as partial shipment poses problems if this amount not available then postpone to any early date. Pls reply."

Krish and I had discussed the significance of a shipment of a lesser number of doses on several occasions. We finally agreed that the original language of Mr. Sharma, the minister of civil aviation, should be adhered to. The following day I sent my last telex (of this visit) to Bill Nurse: "Transportation agreement with the government provides for free shipment for units of 1/2 million doses only. Otherwise accept January 81 delivery for 1/2 million doses. Signed, Ken Hobbs."

We started our return journey from New Delhi, flying to Bangkok. Our six-day stay at the Oriental Hotel, in a top-floor suite, was most enjoyable. We spent most of the time watching the free-flowing traffic on the river. It was amazing to see so many water taxis, ships, barges and boats going in so many different directions all at the same time without any collisions. On a boat trip through the back areas of the river, I was overwhelmed and appalled, watching young children swimming in the grossly polluted water, bathing, cleaning their teeth, and then ending up by drinking a cupful of the polluted water.

We decided to take the train south to Ipoh and then on to Singapore. The Rotary Club of Ipoh, Malaysia, the tin capital of the world, asked me to come and discuss the possibility of setting up a red measles immunization program for them.

The train trip was a never-to-be-forgotten experience. We were unable to purchase tickets for air-conditioned compartments. However, this did not work out badly; the compartment was clean and fairly spacious, and the open windows allowed us to experience the sounds and smells of Thailand and Malaysia.

The highlight of our two-night stay in Ipoh was a wonderful shrimp dinner. We soon learned that not only were the shrimp very large, but the heads were considered a true delicacy and given to the guests of honor as a mark of special favor. Eva and I did make a sincere attempt to follow their custom, with some difficulty.

Our stopover in Kuala Lumpur was uneventful. However, the local Rotarian president was able to secure first class air-conditioned seats for us on our four-hour train ride to Singapore. Some time after our departure from the Kuala Lumpur station, the gentleman sitting across from us struck up a conversation.

"I see that you are a Rotarian."

"Yes, I am," I replied.

"What are you doing in Malaysia?"

I explained why I was there, where we were going, and what we planned to do after we left Singapore. At that, he opened his briefcase, and I realized that he was a real estate salesman.

"You are a Canadian," he remarked, "and it so happens that I have a very valuable, reasonable piece of property listed for sale in Canada." With this he opened his book, and handed me a colored photograph of a building on Elgin Street in Ottawa. It was an office that housed some of the offices of the British High Commission. It is indeed a small world when a Malaysian real estate salesman attempts to sell me an office building in Ottawa, Ontario, on a train travelling from Kuala Lumpur to Singapore.

The arrival in Singapore was uneventful. Descending from the train, we followed the crowd to the inspection station. As we approached the area I became rather concerned: for twenty feet or more, both sides of our four-foot-wide sidewalk were lined with cages crowded with German shepherds in running pens. As I stopped to look in wonder at the dogs the gentleman behind me softly spoke: "If they bark, you are in trouble."

"Why?" I asked.

"Because the dogs are sniffing for illegal drugs," he said, "and if they bark you are in big trouble."

As we approached the inspection station I looked back and watched as a policeman entered the first car of our train with an old German shepherd. Fifteen minutes later I saw them descending from the last railway car. It reminded me of my first visit to Kuala Lumpur in 1979. The first thing you saw on entering the airport for customs and immigration clearance was a large sign that read "All illegal drugs are forbidden in Malaysia. The minimum penalty for conviction is death. You have been warned." I have always thought that this type of sign should be placed in a conspicuous place in all airports in North America. Our stay in the old Raffles Hotel was a pleasure that we will always remember.

During our stay in Hong Kong we had a chance to go back to our two refugee camps for a visit with our friends on the medical staff. It was delightful to see that there were now fewer refugees than six months before during our tour of duty in April and March.

Home was most welcome after this strenuous trip.

Chapter 19

Shortly after our arrival home, Chairman Paul McKelvey called a meeting with the treasurer, myself, and Mr. E.G. O'Hara of Merck, Sharpe and Dohme, regarding the 3.5 million-dose Attenuvax project. Mr. O'Hara confirmed his company's position and their ability to supply the required number of doses of vaccine, but there had apparently been some misunderstanding regarding the price per dose. We were under the impression that it was ten cents US per dose. Mr. O'Hara explained that it was originally quoted at that price by Merck Canada in July 1979; however, no contract had been signed at that time, and the price of the vaccine had risen to fourteen cents US per dose in August 1980. That, he told us, was the price at which they sold the vaccine to U.S. Aid. He further revealed they had an understanding with U.S. Aid that they would not sell to any organization for less than that amount.

A letter of December 8, 1980 outlined Merck, Sharpe and Dohme's position as follows:

> In summary we cannot accept your letter/order of November the 28th, 1980, as issued, and will be able to do so on receipt of your formal acknowledgment of: (1) price is US $0.14 per dose f.o.b. New York; (2) delivery schedule as discussed and previously outlined; (3) your confirmation that you are responsible for air freight beyond the initial 1981 delivery; (4) your confirmation

that you will arrange to obtain an import license amendment if necessary for shipment beyond 2 million doses.

The final agreement was now in place. The committee at its next meeting selected Governor Fran Smith and Past District Governor Obrey Oldham from District 701 to be the first volunteers with the first shipment of vaccine in this expanded red measles immunization program. Rotary International called for two volunteers to accompany each shipment of vaccine.

In early December I received a letter from New Delhi, dated November 15. The writer was none other than Henricus W. H. Lucker, officer in charge of UNICEF India. He was responding to the letter I had sent him from Madras on October 15. He relayed the following:

> As was suggested in your letter of 15th October 1980, the matter has been taken up with the Ministry of Health & Family Welfare, Government of India, and specifically the draft "hold harmless" agreement which should be signed by the government for the scheduled supply of measles vaccine over the period of three years.
>
> Unfortunately the government cannot accept the clause of the draft agreement wherein Rotary International disclaims any guarantee or warranty of any kind, expressed or implied, with respect to the quality, fitness or merchantability of vaccines, purchased or donated, supplied to the ministry of health. The reasons for ministry's unacceptance are:
>
> 1) It presently conducts with "WHO" technical guidance, feasibility on introduction of mass immunization against measles in the country and therefore pays particular attention to the quality, fitness and merchantability of vaccines being supplied for the study. 2) The study is to be continued for two years more since 25 medical col-

leges are involved in it. The government will need the entire lot of measles vaccines each year at specified dates. 3) The vaccine should have adequate refrigeration facilities at Bombay at the Central Research Institute, Kasauli (H.P.). 4) The delivery dates shown in your letter do not correspond to the ministerial requirements.

We very much appreciate the kind offer of Rotary International to provide the vaccine for the feasibility study and regret, due to the reasons given above, it will not be possible to accept your offer at this time.

With kind regards, Yours sincerely, Henricus W. H. Lucker, Officer in Charge, UNICEF India

The year could not end without another confrontation. John Stucky called me on December 29, 1980, stating that a medical member of Rotary's 3H committee had phoned him, complaining about the lack of Rotary promotion in our 68,000-dose initial red measles immunization program in India. After a lengthy discussion without any names being mentioned, we wished each other a happy New Year and ended our phone conversation.

I followed up that conversation with a letter to John Stucky, dated December 29, 1980. The essential communication was as follows:

> Further to our telephone conversation today, I might add that I was very upset that a member of the 3H Committee would make such a foolish statement as that Rotary and in particular Rotary International was either neglected or overlooked in the publicity for the expanded program of immunization against measles, which was started in a modest way by District 707 in 1979.
>
> Over the past fifteen months my wife and I have spent six months in international service. I might add that this has been at our own expense except for my airfare to

Hong Kong and $200 a week for our living accommodations at the YMCA in Kowloon. Not one other penny did I ask for or intend to receive either from my home club, District 707 or Rotary International. As a modest cost I would estimate my personal involvement, through loss of income and travel expenses to be in the neighborhood of $50,000. I have always attempted to live up to the ideals of Rotary. I have always been able to answer in the affirmative to the four-way test to any of my actions in Canada, India or Hong Kong.

I have always considered myself to be a positive individual and find it difficult to deal with negative people—especially negative Rotarians when it applies to World Community Service or the basic principles of the 3H program. It amazes me that a member of your committee would contact a person in Vellore and complain that Rotary International and the 3H program were not paramount in the publicity given this expanded program, when indeed the first shipment in this expanded program will not arrive in India for at least another four weeks.

Enclosed are a few copies of some of the publicity regarding Rotary International's involvement in Districts 320 and 321. Once again I would urge you, John, to visit these districts and see for yourself. Perhaps this "Rotarian" will have the opportunity to visit South India. He will then be in a position to be able to publish an unbiased and stimulating article on the significance of Rotary International's meaningful involvement in this program. Yours in Rotary, for a better world, Ken Hobbs MD.

Thus another year ended.

Chapter 20

The early part of January 1981 was spent communicating via telex with Krish Chitale and Merck, Sharpe and Dohme, in an attempt to crystallize the shipping date. There was some confusion between Air India and Mr. O'Hara of Merck, Sharpe and Dohme. This was finally settled, and I sent the following telex to Krish on January 15, 1981:

> Vaccine leaves January 17 Air India Flight 190 Arrives Bombay 05:35 January 19. Departs Bombay India Air 191 19:15 January 19. Arrives Madras January 20 02:05. Will require 14 hour storage while in Bombay. Air bill number 098-31619556, 45 or 46 pieces. Weight 5300 lb.. Smith and Oldham arrive Madras Air India 439 Jan 21 09:55 Notify G.V. and Ramesh: Ken Hobbs, MD.

I looked forward to Krish's next telex, which was sent from Madras on 20 January:

> Reproducing copy of telex sent to JJ Lauria Merck Sharpe and Dohme international. Consignment arrived last night intact. Many thanks for all the help. Governors arrived Delhi this morning. Appointments fixed as scheduled in Delhi. Reaching Madras tomorrow. Chitale.

The impossible dream was now a reality. Half a million doses of red measles vaccine were stored in cold lockers in Madras. Our past difficulties now looked minuscule. The door was open to advance our dream of eradicating measles in South India. I say our dream, but by that I mean the never-ending dream that Krish and I had entertained since our first meeting, on September 15, 1979.

Governor Fran Smith of Scarborough telexed me his news of the project on January 23, 1980:

> Vaccine unpacked OK. Stored in King Institute. Met with press and doctors yesterday, also president Madras Club. First draw on shipment to Vellore same day via Dr. John. All scheduled appointments Delhi made. Chitale wonderful host. Your good work very evident. Attended reception with minister of health and top medical people. Interviewed by press and TV. Regards, Fran.

The last difficulty—that insurmountable mountain concerning the lack of Rotary International publicity in our pilot project—still remained. John Stucky, however, was becoming a believer. In a letter to me on January 13, he stated:

> Dear Ken: Thank you for burying me in clippings, Rotary bulletins, and your letter expressing amazement that anyone would ever have lost sight or failed to hear that the red measles program in India is a Rotary International Health, Hunger, and Humanity Program project. Ken, I personally appreciate how hard you have worked with Dr. Jacob John and numerous Indian Rotarians. The 3H program needs more Rotarians like those in the measles program, who will go through all the steps to bring such projects from the idea stage to

reality. Thank you, John Stucky (manager, Health, Hunger, and Humanity Program).

Janet Long, John Stucky's assistant, sent an information letter to a Mr. Michael H. Anderson, information officer for UNICEF in New York. I quote from her letter:

> I have enclosed two press clippings concerning red measles vaccination project in Southern India, apparently the first in the country. Dr. Ken Hobbs, who was instrumental in organizing and implementing this project, talked with an Indian physician who was researching the causes of blindness among children in his area. He is convinced that as much as 20 percent is caused by measles. I am sure that Dr. Hobbs would be happy to talk with you regarding specific details. His phone number is listed on the press release.

Mim Neal of the public relations office of Rotary International issued the first press release to all of the newspapers in Canada. The headline was "Rotary International initiates red measles immunization in India. First 500,000 vaccines to be sent to Madras." The release then covered a brief history and the present approved 3.5 million-dose project.

The problem of the conversation that I had had with John Stucky was still not resolved. However, I did receive a letter, written on January 16, from a Rotarian, Dr. John Sever. In his letter he mentions the visit of one of his colleagues, a Dr. Madden, to Vellore, and his talk regarding Dr. Jacob John's interest in and use of measles vaccine. Then the mystery started to unravel.

In a letter dated February 6, 1981, Dr. Jacob John related to John Stucky that he had met Dr. David Madden and discussed his interest in the red measles immunization program. He also related to John Stucky that he had received a phone call from the USA, from Dr. Sever. I now quote from Dr. Jacob John's letter to John Stucky of February 6, 1981.

> ...I happened to mention to him the importance of red measles immunization in South India. I had not realized that he (Dr. John Sever) was interested in Rotary, and I am sure that he did not realize that I was a Rotarian. Thus I might have been instrumental in creating an impression in Dr. Sever's mind that the measles immunization program conducted by the department of virology was a program of the Christian Medical College Hospital at Vellore. In fact this program has very little to do with the Medical College Hospital, except that I work here, and that I have used institutional facilities to push the program in Vellore town. The public in South India have come to understand measles vaccine and Rotary as almost synonymous.
>
> You might be interested to know that the entire program was based in the community and not through the normal channels of Christian Medical College Hospital. This decision was made by me at the very start. My co-Rotarians did not understand why I insisted that we should give no room for anyone to suspect that this program was being pushed by any other institution than the Rotary clubs of South India...for the first time in our club's history, the Vellore Club has given me a citation for promoting the cause of Rotary, through the measles immunization program...
>
> The district officials and members of my own club are in no doubt that my work in measles immunization is accomplished wearing a Rotary hat, and not the CMCH hat. If I did not make it clear to Dr. Sever, I now apologize for my oversight. I would like to state categorically

that there need be no more apprehension that the Rotary's role is underplayed in South India. The impact that Rotary has made in the last year in South India is something to be proud of by every Rotarian all over the world. I trust that this matter could be laid to rest and our attention, time and resources could be fully utilized for service under the 3H program of Rotary International. With kind regards, Yours sincerely, Rtn. T. Jacob John, Department of Virology, CMC Hospital, Vellore, 632 004 India.

A congratulatory letter was sent to Krish Chitale in early March 1981 by John Stucky:

Dear Krish: Ken Hobbs' reports on the India measles project have been very exciting. We all look forward to each progress report of this project and wish other countries' involvement of Rotarians would be as effective. Ken has made it clear that your untiring efforts have made the project possible. Without your work behind the scenes, progress might have been stopped in the earliest stages. I am sure you derive special personal satisfaction in watching this project unfold, but please know how very much your efforts are appreciated by the 3H program. Thank you and congratulations for the significant success you brought to the measles immunization program. Sincerely, John Stucky, manager, Health, Hunger, and Humanity Program.

Herb Pigman, the General Secretary of Rotary International, had forwarded me a copy of a letter from a Rotarian I had never met. In the Rotarian's letter, Rotarian P.V. Puroshothaman, better known as "Puro," reported that the clubs in the immediate Salem (South India) area had

· Diary of a Miracle ·

gone beyond the 60,000-dose allotment and were expecting to immunize 150,000 children by the end of April 1981. He further pointed out that this amount exceeded the original target by 800 percent. He enclosed several photos of the red measles camps conducted in the Salem area.

General Secretary Herb Pigman sent letters of congratulation to the president of each of the ten Rotary clubs that were involved in this tremendous display of "service above self." He wrote that

> ...the achievement of ten Rotary clubs in immunizing more than 150,000 children, between 15 March and 15 May 1981 is truly impressive. The Rotary club of Namakkal, which is under your able leadership, was responsible for 4,650 immunizations, and played an important role in this significant accomplishment. A generation of children in Tamil Nadu and Kerala will have you to thank for your part in freeing them from blindness, deafness, brain damage, and needless deaths. Rotary International congratulates you and extends to you a deep appreciation for your humanitarian service.

This letter also went out to President R. Muthiah of the Salem club; President A.R. Mudaliar of the Rotary Club of Tiruchengode; President Dr. R.Subramaniam of the Rotary Club of Salem West; President M.H. Mehta of the Rotary Club of Salem North; President K.S.S. Raghavan of the Rotary Club of Mettur Dam; President P.S. George of the Rotary Club of Erode; President Raju Jagannathan of the Rotary Club of Dharmpauiri; President A.M.V. Jayaraman of the Rotary Club of Bhavani.

Herb Pigman's thank-you letter to Puro was as follows:

> Thank you for your excellent letter and report. The achievement of ten Rotary clubs in immunizing more than 150,000 children against measles between 15

March and the 15th May, 1981, is truly impressive. The Rotary club of Salem Mid-town, which under your able leadership was responsible for immunizing 78,080 children, played an important role in this significant accomplishment.

In mid-June my attention turned to getting everything in order for the September shipment. The essential factor was receiving the approval for free shipment by Air India. Each shipment was independently approved by the civil aviation authorities. I sent this telex to Krish on June 24: "Require Air India approval free shipments September. Ken Hobbs."

The following day Krish sent me this reply: "Received telex. Just received free shipment approval for 500,000 doses to reach here before 30th November (copy of this telex sent to John Stucky). Chitale."

The two volunteers to accompany the shipment of 500,000 doses of measles vaccine had been chosen: Past District Governor Dave Theunissen from Swan Lake, Manitoba, and Alex Clough from Australia. The necessary agenda in India was handled by Krish as usual. I kept him informed as to when and how they would be arriving in Madras.

I had been chosen by our district to lead a GSE team to District 320 in January 1982. (A GSE team is a group study exchange team; this is a program sponsored by The Rotary Foundation. The team consists of a Rotarian leader and five non-Rotarians between the ages of twenty-five and thirty-five. The team visits another district in the Rotary world and spends a minimum of five weeks visiting, living with the local Rotarians and gaining a first-hand knowledge of the local customs and culture.) I had the good fortune to be chosen as leader, as this was the district that I had visited twice before: first in 1979 in the original pilot red measles program and then in the initial expanded phase of the 3.5-million-dose program. The team's plan was to arrive in Madras on December 31, 1982, after visiting Agra and the Taj Mahal, compliments of one of Krish Chitale's friends.

On September 22, Chairman Paul McKelvey received the following telex: "Measles vaccine arrived yesterday in good condition, regards, Dave Theunissen."

Another success story. The second shipment arrived. However, I was worried. How many doses were still left from the first shipment? This was one of the questions I had asked Krish in one of my communications, but he had avoided answering this important question. I knew that I would be in Madras and South India for six weeks beginning on the 31st of December.

In one of our many telephone conversations with John Stucky, the question of our possible involvement in programs and projects in Africa (Eva's and mine) was raised. We had made a firm decision: we were available. This was conveyed to John Stucky on numerous occasions. I assured him that there would be no cost to Rotary International. Once we had made our first decision to donate our services to the Indian red measles project, the precedent had been set. Wherever we go on behalf of Rotary, there will be no cost to Rotary International.

In mid-July 1981, John Stucky asked us to travel, as the special representatives of Rotary International President Stan McCaffrey, to four West African countries: Senegal, the Gambia, Sierra Leone and Morocco. The purpose of the visit was to provide assistance and stimulation to local Rotarians who wished to initiate a 3H application for a polio program in their countries.

Eva and I went to Evanston at the end of August for a briefing session. This gave me the opportunity of meeting John Stucky again, and perhaps more important, meeting his staff: Sarah Cook, Janet Long and Mim Neal. These three young women were indeed a tremendous asset to Rotary International. (Only Mim Neal remains in their employment). A debriefing session was held on our return. President Stan McCaffery came to John Stucky's small cubicle when he heard that Eva and I were at 1400 Ridge Avenue. He personally thanked us and expressed his gratitude for our endeavors.

We arrived in Dakar, Senegal, at 3:30 a.m. on September 15, 1981. A tired, sleepy-eyed Rotarian by the name of Jean Desplaits met us at the airport and assisted us in clearing immigration and customs. On our way into the city we were unexpectedly stopped by armed policemen, who insisted that I open all of our luggage. A thorough search was carried out under flashlight illumination. This was certainly a new experience. We had nothing to hide, or be worried about, but my cardiac rate did increase to over 180 beats per minute. This would be the first of our many remarkable and unusual experiences in Senegal.

The UNICEF officer was very cooperative. The Rotarians were receptive to the idea of instituting a polio program. The health officials, on the other hand, were reserved and uncommunicative. The Rotarians showed us the highlights of Dakar, including Gore Island, where we saw the small hole in the wall of the fort, through which most of the slave trade victims passed in the late 1700s and early 1800s.

We also met a most remarkable man, who had dedicated his life to helping crippled children in the Dakar area. It was a very warm and humid morning when the Rotarians took Eva and me to his training center. As we entered his room, a strong smell of urine met us. A very small, bearded gentleman was lying covered up in bed. He had an obvious physical problem, and appeared grotesque. However, the exact etiology of his condition would have been difficult to diagnose. I did not feel comfortable inquiring about the nature of his physical problems, especially with the Rotarians present.

The bed had hand bars, which enabled him to raise and lower himself when he was lying in his bed. After a short conversation in French, the Rotarians told me that he was in charge of a training center for the rehabilitation of polio victims. With a charming smile on his pleasant face, he invited me to visit his brace manufacturing center. Before we left him, I asked if he would permit me to take his picture.

He quickly responded, in French, "No, doctor, because if your people see my photograph they will feel sorry for me. I do not feel sorry for myself. You and your friends must always feel sorry for the children who cannot walk." His words resound in my memory every time a see a "polio crawler." However, he did consent to my taking his picture, conditional upon my promise that I would always remember the children who required help in walking.

We visited his brace center. I was appalled at the antiquated method used in hammering out the brace material. I was told it would take approximately two weeks for a technician to make one brace; this was the usual, accepted method. The brace was forged out of raw steel over a fire, using techniques similar to those of an old-fashioned blacksmith. The same method was used in the other three West African countries we would visit.

On my return to Canada I formulated a plan for a "West African brace project," to help the four countries develop modern brace-making techniques. The total budget was $450,000, of which $70,000 was raised in District 7070, the remainder from CIDA and the Rotary International 3H funding program.

A local Rotarian (a pharmacist) flew us to Banjul in the Gambia in his personal six-seater Cessna. There had been a recent coup in the Gambia, and most airlines were not flying into Banjul.

In the Gambia we saw the same method of brace-making. A new Rotary club had recently been chartered and they were very positive about the idea of a polio immunization project.

In Freetown, Sierra Leone, we were confronted immediately after landing by an immigration officer who told us that since we did not have an entry visa, we also did not have an exit visa. We were informed that these must be secured immediately at their downtown office. Downtown, it transpired, was some thirty-five miles away over dusty roads, plus a one-hour trip on the local ferry. The Rotarians sent a young man to pick us up at the airport. Without his help and guidance we would not have been allowed to leave the airport.

Our guide took us to a government office. After much confusion, we ended up in the income tax office. We needed an income-tax clearance before they would grant us entry and exit visas. This took approximately two hours, and in the end, for $25 (US) more than the official cost of the visa, it was issued. The young man was apologetic about asking for the extra money, but I had learned that this is the way business is done in most parts of the developing world.

Across the street from the income tax office was a travel agency. Thinking that it might be a good idea to reconfirm our tickets, I went in, and was told that the flight we were booked on no longer existed! I would have to purchase new tickets in order to be able to leave the country. The tickets were made up, and I presented my American Express card. The young lady took it and disappeared into the back room. Ten minutes later, a short, bald, and rather obese young man, who appeared to be of Lebanese origin, emerged.

"Your American Express card is not in order. It expires in thirty days. I am sorry, we cannot accept it for payment of your tickets. Do you have another credit card?"

When I said I had no other card, he beckoned me to come into the back room, where, after considerable persuasion, he agreed to accept the payment by American Express if I consented to pay an extra fifty dollars. We left the travel agency with our tickets. The young man, our guide, then drove us to the large hotel by the central banyan tree.

At the hotel a delegation of Rotarians, who had been waiting to greet us, swarmed our guide, vehemently criticizing the young man for being three and half hours late. Eventually I was able to get their attention and explain that our lateness was not his fault, but mine. The misunderstanding was soon sorted out, and we were escorted to the home of our hosts Suru Davies and his wife Tunde, with whom we had an exceptionally pleasant stay in Freetown.

Later that afternoon I had the pleasure of meeting the US ambassador, an African-American lady. We discussed the proposed polio project at length. At the end of our conversation, the ambassador turned to me and said, "Dr. Hobbs, do you realize that one of a woman's major responsibilities, twice every day, is walking some three miles to fetch water? Hopefully, Rotary will perhaps some day be able to help these women by discovering and creating clean water sources, near where they live."

I have never forgotten her forceful and heartfelt words. Wherever I travel in the developing world, when I see women carrying children in their arms and water casks on their heads, I hear again the American ambassador to Sierra Leone, on that sunny warm afternoon in 1981 in Freetown.

Before we left Freetown, a tentative 3H application had been endorsed by the Rotarians, and that made up for the frustrations we had experienced on arrival.

Late one evening, four days later, we were met in Casablanca by a Rabat Rotarian. My stay in Rabat was consumed by long negotiations with health ministry officials. The discussions, all in French, went on for three days, as I attempted to obtain their endorsement of a $1,000,000 Rotary International polio project. It was difficult, to say the least. The last hours of negotiation were very stressful, but suddenly the meeting ended, and we were joined by the minister of health and surrounded by TV cameras. On live TV, the minister announced the successful conclusion of our three days of complicated negotiations.

Our work in West Africa, which began in mid-September in Senegal and ended three weeks later in Morocco, was very successful. My French had been good enough to consummate an agreement for our largest immunization project of all, a one-million-dollar (in US funds) polio project in Morocco. Eva and I would make many more trips to Africa in the future on behalf on Rotary International.

Our return home brought me back to the reality of our measles project. Our next two volunteers were chosen to accompany the shipment in January 1982; they were past District Governor Jack Laycock from St. Stephen, New Brunswick, and Rotarian Teddy Yamada from Japan. They would be the last of the non-committee volunteers. There were two reasons for this decision. First, the volunteers who had not been committee members were not conversant with the project's basic premise and guidelines. This had inadvertently caused confusion for Krish's committee in Madras. Second, they attempted to go beyond the criteria originally laid down for the performance of the project. My suggestion that in future only committee members act as volunteers, which I made in my report following my January 1982 visit, was endorsed by the committee.

As December approached, the necessary agreements for the shipment of measles vaccine to India had to be finalized. I was once again aghast when I received the following familiar telex from Krish, on December 14,1981: "Strongly suggest postponement of 3rd allotment till you arrive. Facing approval problems and uptake of vaccine from the district. Chitale."

As I prepared to leave Canada on December 26, 1981, with my group study exchange team for District 320 South India, I couldn't help hoping that perhaps just one shipment of vaccine would go tickety-boo, without any problems.

Chapter 21

On our arrival in Madras on December 31, 1981, our welcome was as punctilious and festive as usual. Krish arranged a gathering of Rotarians to meet the GSE team later on in the evening, but, more important, he gathered together a core group of Rotarians from the district who were committed, hard-working advocates of the measles project.

One of these advocates was "Puro." He and I had exchanged letters, but never met. Puro was a strong, positive, assertive individual, who left a lasting impression on my memory; he spoke in such a way as to instantly capture your attention and keep you mesmerized. After a thirty-minute conversation with Puro, I felt completely assured that nothing would sidetrack our immunization project. He was indeed an organizer, and highly practical, and had a discreet way of inspiring confidence. His concern for the maintenance of the "cold chain" was refreshing. As I look back on that conversation, I can see that even then it was clear that he intended to revolutionize cold chain methodology and service training maintenance for any immunization program in the future. These reforms came to fruition during the polio immunization project sponsored by our club (the Rotary Club of Whitby, Ontario) and approved by The Rotary Foundation in June 1985.

Once again there was confusion over the free air shipment of the vaccine. A telex to Bill Nurse from Krish dated January 16, 1982, stated: "Civil aviation instructions to Air India posted on 29th December. Reference No. AV 13020/76/80A dated December 15, 1981. Posting one more copy with import permit today. Pls give correct flight and names of Rotarians arriving January 18. Chitale."

· Madras: December 1981, 1982, 1983 ·

On January 21, 1982, Bill Nurse notified Krish by telex: "Free carriage received revised shipping schedule arrive Madras Air India 424 January 28 0.910. Concerned about connection in Bombay. Please monitor. Mckelvey."

Fortunately, my GSE team arrived back in Madras the morning of January 28, in time to witness the arrival and unloading of the vaccine. As I stood on the tarmac, the sound of the unloading of the 500,000 doses of vaccine by the tractors and other equipment was music to my ears. Viewing the vaccine packed in its heat-impregnable containers made me very proud to be a Rotarian.

We accompanied the vaccine to the King Institute, the research and storage facility for all the perishable vaccines for the state of Tamil Nadu. Their controlled atmospheric environment was excellent. The unpacking of the containers was very satisfactory: even though the vaccine had been in transit from New York City for some ninety-six hours, the content of the containers was still frozen solid.

I sent the following telex to Bill Nurse: "Vaccine arrived in good condition. Inform McKelvey notify O'Hara inform Eva. Will phone February 8th a.m. Team are all well. Ken."

The GSE team had spent the previous four weeks in India and had become familiar with the immunization project and the effect it had on the Rotarians of South India. However, there were now some new and alarming problems. The Rotarians were becoming fatigued with their responsibilities.

That evening, Krish and I had a heart-to-heart talk. The question we asked each other was, where do we go from here? Up to this point, the Rotarians had single-handedly immunized two and a half million children against red measles, and our troops were tiring. We had proven beyond a shadow of a doubt that the program was justified and successful. Rotary, however, was not really in the health business, and the ministry of health of the state of Tamil Nadu was. I suggested that I would like to have a meeting with the minister of health, Dr. Hande (whom I had met on my previous trip to South India), to discuss the responsibilities of the ministry. The minister's help was required now. I suggested that a meeting be convened as soon as possible. Two days later, the minister called a meeting in his office.

At the meeting, I asked for government support and help in completing the project. I outlined what I thought would be the perfect solution: a combined ministry of health and Rotary committee to oversee and supervise the red measles immunization program. I also pointed out that our past experience with certain officials had not been productive, in that they could not make a decision and were apt to change their minds even after they seemed to have arrived at a definite conclusion.

The minister said: "Dr. Hobbs, that problem is now solved. Gathered here are my senior advisers." With that, he turned to them and said: "You have heard the good doctor. I do not want to hear of any disagreement with the Rotarians on this committee. If there is, I would ask Mr. Chitale to approach me personally. If that happens then I will deal with both the problem and the matter of your personal usefulness to me as minister of health, do you understand?"

All the government officials nodded in unison. That meeting was the breakthrough in the relationship between Rotary International and the government of Tamil Nadu. I feel that Dr. Hande's attitude and accomplishment set a precedent in the developing world, as far as goodwill and communications between our organization and the developing world's government bureaucracy were concerned.

A committee of Rotarians and government officials was formed. Dr. Hande stipulated to his officials that they must cooperate with Rotary and make their own direct and positive decisions. This was indeed the turning point of the red measles immunization project. The state government was now moving forward.

On March 6, 1982, Krish Chitale wrote to John Stucky: "We have now obtained a hold harmless agreement from the government of Tamil Nadu in respect of all immunological agencies including measles vaccine and a Xerox copy of the agreement is enclosed for your reference.

I hope this helps in obtaining other vaccines also through RI's 3H program."

On April 15, the secretary of the measles committee for District 320 wrote and suggested that they would request that from now on we send only one volunteer per shipment. This was endorsed by our committee, who also agreed that the volunteer should be one of themselves. In this way we could ensure that the volunteer would be a knowledgeable person, rather than a person who, however well-meaning, would have had no direct experience with the project.

In April of 1982, I received a delightful, informative letter from Puro, and I quote from sections of his letter:

> I am extremely happy to inform you that we have set a stage for liquidating all the stock from the King Institute, Madras before the end of May, perhaps the district may run dry of measles vaccine by August '82…I understand Chingleput District is going ahead for immunizing 100,000. Dharmapuri District will be immunizing 125,000 and Periyar District will be immunizing 125,000. With this achievement before the end of May, there will be very little vaccine left over…I have printed a guideline for the measles immunization programme and I am enclosing a copy for your reference.

Another communication reached me at about this time, of a very different nature. Krish forwarded a copy of the newspaper *The Hindu*, dated May 9, 1982. The news was tragic. Two children had died from receiving measles vaccine and another twenty-seven were very ill. An immediate follow-up of these deaths by Dr. Jacob John discovered that vaccine left in a partially used 50-dose vial had been administered. This was contrary to the written acceptable procedure designed by himself. The 50 ml vial of vaccine should have been destroyed, but instead it was left unrefrigerated for several days, then used to vaccinate twenty-nine children, in order to use up the vaccine. Twenty minutes after their immunization, all of the children fell ill. A local doctor had the presence of mind to save the vial and turn it over to Dr. Jacob John. Cultures of the remaining contents in the vial revealed the presence of staphylococcus aureus, a deadly bacterial contamination. This bacteria produces a toxin that is known to cause vomiting, diarrhea and dehydration, which may lead to death in children if immediate medical care is not given.

The newspaper article went on to report:

> Dr. Jacob John received a communication from a Rotarian in Salem, along with the used vial. According to the letter the camps were conducted on April 30 in Thalaivaipalayam Village, by two teams of doctors. One team immunized the children of the village while the second team immunized only children of the local elementary school. Out of the 104 children immunized in the school, twenty-five developed vomiting, diarrhea and dehydration eight hours after immunization. In the evening one child, aged four, died; another child, aged one and a half, died after being taken to hospital at Tirupur. The other twenty-five children were admitted at Erode and Tirupur and they are reported to be progressing.

According to the newspaper, children of the village immunized by the first team had no reaction whatsoever. Dr. Jacob John said that in North Arcot District, 1.5 *lakh* (the Indian word for the number 100,000; 1.5 *lakh* equals 150,000, or written in the Indian manner, 1,50,000) immunizations had been given so far without a single report of reaction or ill effects. He suggested that those supervising the mass immunization program should take proper care with respect to sterilization of equipment and the safe cold storage of vaccine to avert reactions.

This article was published right after this catastrophic episode. Dr.

· *Madras: December 1981, 1982, 1983* ·

Jacob John's quick response was crucial in salvaging the people's faith in the red measles immunization program in this important area of the state of Tamil Nadu.

Krish also forwarded an updated report of the distribution of the vaccine on June 1, 1982. It was as follows:

District 320

1) Vellore 1,44,000
2) Coimbatore, Goup Otacamund, Tripur, Gudalur, Mettupalayam, Udumalpet, Palaghat 1,33,000
3) Tanjore 50,800
4) Cochin 50,000
5) Trichur 24,000
6) Institute of Child Health and Madras ..1,34,000
7) Cuddalore 6,000
8) Calicut 48,000
9) Salem Group, (Mettur Dam, Erode, Dharmapuri, Bhavani, Gopichetty Palayam, Sathamangalam and Salem Clubs) 4,200,400
10) Kodugallur 4,800
11) Pennnadam 1,200
12) Kumbakonam 13,200
13) Nagapattinam 7,200
14) Chidambaram 2,400

District 321 13,27,200

1) Trivandrum 48,000
2) Kottayam 72,000
3) Madurai 1,20,000

4) Trichy 48,000
   Balance on date (doses): 2,41,600

Total doses received (including pilot project): 15,68,60

The committee's next volunteer was PDG Wilf Wilkinson, who acted as the treasurer for both phases of the measles vaccine project. This was his first visit to India. Wilf was scheduled to leave for India on the September 8 and return on October 2. The shipment of 500,000 doses of measles vaccine was scheduled to arrive in Madras on September 30. However, the exact date of shipment was not definitely confirmed until the last moment.

Puro kept his group in Salem very active. His letter of September 20 was intensely positive. He reported:

> I am extremely happy to inform you that we have celebrated the crossing of the 500,000 mark of doses of vaccine given by our group IV consisting of 11 clubs of Salem on the 17th of September....You will also be happy to learn that we have completely exhausted the 1.5 million doses measles vaccine so far supplied to districts 320 and 321. We are eagerly awaiting the arrival of the fourth consignment of 500,000 doses during the first week of October '82.

The program was now under way in earnest. A press clipping from *The Hindu* of September 24, 1982, declared:

> In the early stages the measles immunization program left much to be desired as the private medical practitioners could not devote their full time to the project and complementary support from governmental institutions was not forthcoming. In fact at one stage, Dr. Ken Hobbs,

Madras: December 1981, 1982, 1983

known as the 'father of the anti-measles vaccine campaign,' who was instrumental in getting the project for Tamil Nadu, persuaded Dr. Hande the Minister of Health to endorse and help in the campaign with the help of the health departments and all the local district collectors of the state. Already two million doses of the vaccine have been received and used in all districts of the state.

The year ended on an up note. The next two volunteers would be Rotarian Dr. John Severs and District Governor Fred Black. They were preparing for their January 1983 visit.

I was preparing to go to Medan, Sumatra, Indonesia, on February 25, 1983, on a 3H project involving the Methodist Church and Rotary International. I would be the first medical doctor, along with a dentist from California, to be assigned as a 100-percent volunteer to this project. We would be going on a reconverted fifty-foot fishing vessel to the swamp islands off Singapore to administer medical and dental care to these isolated natives who had never before seen a doctor or a dentist.

Unfortunately, after waiting six weeks for the vessel to be prepared, we were refused permission to leave port by the government authorities, due to their fear of the Methodist Church's role in converting natives in these areas.

Chapter 22

PDG John Severs and PDG Fred Black witnessed the arrival of 500,000 doses of red measles vaccine in Madras at the end of January 1983. Dr. Severs is a prominent virologist working for US CDC Atlanta, with his offices in Washington, DC. His report was very thorough and informative. The following are excerpts from his report:

> Measles immunization is being carried on by private physicians in India. About 100,000 doses are used each year. The vaccine is now available free of customs duty at a cost of 3 rupees (about $.30) per dose. The government does not have an national policy concerning measles immunization. Vaccines which are provided by the government include DPT, BCG and polio.
>
> There are two measles immunization programs now in progress:
>
> 1) the Rotary-CIDA project in two southern states of Tamil Nadu and Kerala, and
>
> 2) the measles immunization project (study) of the EPI [expanded program for immunization] section of the directorate general health services, New Delhi which is being carried out in 28 medical centers. Both programs should be completed in about a year.

This project in Tamil Nadu and Kerala was initiated in 1979 under the medical direction of Dr. Jacob John, an internationally known pediatrician-virologist at the Christian Medical College, Vellore, Rotarian Krish Chitale of Madras, India, and Rotarian Dr. Kenneth Hobbs of Ontario, Canada, are key individuals in this project ... Cold chain distribution has been through volunteer Rotarians and has been excellent...

In conjunction with this project Dr. Jacob John is preparing several reports:

1) "Conduct of a successful mass measles immunization program in India": a medical publication which will describe how this successful program was accomplished. The planning and completion data should help other areas in developing similar programs. Dr. John will write the draft of this paper and collaborators will contribute.

2) "Antibody response to measles vaccine in a mass campaign." A medical publication is being prepared on the serological findings following the use of the present vaccine in Vellore. Data is already available and Dr. John is preparing his paper.

3) "Complications occurring in a mass measles immunization program." A report to WHO in New Delhi on the three episodes of illness. Two associated with deaths which occurred in the present campaign. These unfortunate events appear to be related to inappropriate use of contaminated vaccine that was kept for days at room temperature and then given.

These isolated problems were caused by rare individuals failing to adhere to clear directions covering the use of the vaccine. Dr. John will write a report to WHO-New Delhi on these problems and the actions to prevent recurrences. He has already reported these episodes to the state health authorities, the federal health authorities in Delhi (Dr. Basu) and the WHO in Geneva-EPI (Dr. Henderson).

4) "Immune response to measles vaccine in the field." This would be a new study and is under consideration. It would consist of two approaches: A) Antibody responses in 200 children in field conditions of vaccine administration. B) Testing of 10 different samples of vaccine brought back from field use. Part A would show value of vaccine under actual field use. Part B would show potency of the vaccine which had actually been used in the field. Dr. John is considering these studies. Part A would require getting bloods in the field. Part B would be easy but would not demonstrate effect of the vaccine.

5) "Conduct of 'camps' for measles vaccine."

6) Excerpts from newspaper articles on measles vaccine: "There is no government support for measles immunization. All vaccine is imported"..."the government has been contacted by two firms concerning a 'technology transfer'"..."Dr. Ziegler discussed the Rotary-CIDA measles vaccine project in southern India. He knew of this effort through Dr. Jacob John and felt the project was full of enthusiasm and activ-

ity. Unfortunately, the project is not part of the multi-center study being done by Dr. Basu. ..."WHO has seen no reports or publications from the Rotary-CIDA program. He told me of newspaper reports of illness in 30 children and at least one death after receiving contaminated vaccine from the project"...

Dr. Sever concluded his report with a personal letter to Chairman Paul, in which he suggested, "I think we should approach Rotary international immediately to give a special award to Ken Hobbs, and others in 707, as well as Jacob John and Krish Chitale of 320 at the International meeting in Toronto for their outstanding work in this project."

In January 1983, John Stucky of Rotary International asked me to be the first 100-percent medical volunteer to a 3H project in Sumatra, Indonesia. (A 100-percent volunteer is one who receives no compensation from Rotary International. I was the first medical doctor to donate my services in this manner.)

As mentioned in the last chapter, the project was composed of two parts. The first was the outfitting of a fifty-foot motorized vessel by the Methodist Church. Rotary International was allocating $100,000 (US) to equip the vessel with medical and dental instruments and supplies, and would provide medical and dental expertise for a minimum of six to eight weeks per volunteer over a five-year period. Rotary International anticipated that they would have no difficulty in securing volunteers year-round. The second part of the project was the setting up of an agricultural education center and farm some one hundred miles outside of Medan. At the farm, a Rotary volunteer from Holland taught the basics of crop rotation, the raising of rabbits for food, the establishment of a poultry industry, etc. Eighteen students would be enrolled for a six-month session. The rotation of students was scheduled to go on for five years.

I would sail on the equipped vessel from Medan on the northern tip of the island of Sumatra to the Swamp Islands off Singapore, where the medical team, myself and one dentist, would provide medical and dental services to a group of people who had never had access to them before.

Eva and I flew out of Toronto on the 20th of February. We had a ten-day stopover in Tokyo. We managed to see a little of the country, including a visit to Hiroshima. We were amazed to find the city green, with impressive, tall trees. The Remembrance Museum was a lifetime of impressions. We will never forget the silhouettes of human beings burnt in pieces of massive stone and sections of concrete; they are imprinted on our subconscious minds forever.

Our arrival in Medan was unheralded. We were met by an elderly Methodist missionary from the US, the Reverend Leslie Day. Rev. Day was a kind, thoughtful, understanding individual. We were housed at the Methodist compound, the home of the bishop. Also living in the compound was another American missionary, Fred Ingold and his wife, Polly, who was a physiotherapist at the hospital. She was my contact when we were ordering and purchasing medical equipment and supplies for the vessel, named *Anugra*. Both Fred and Leslie had been inducted into the newly chartered Rotary Club of Medan.

Part of the package deal for living in the compound was breakfast with the bishop and his wife. Sharp at 7:00 a.m., we would sit down. The cook would immediately place our breakfast of two fried eggs, sunny side up, before us, and the bishop would commence his morning prayers. This ceremony was familiar to me: my mother had been a Methodist before the formation of the United Church of Canada, and from an early age I had been exposed to the saying of grace and lengthy prayers before each and every meal.

The bishop's eloquence at prayer gave me plenty of time to study the food before we began to eat. On gazing down at my eggs on the first morning, I observed that houseflies were busy attempting to consume my breakfast. I also noticed, much to my shock, that the eggs had a putrid green tinge, due to the grease they had been cooked in. Every morning after that, I discreetly waved both hands over my plate of eggs while the bishop was saying his prayers and blessings, to frighten off the flies. This became a ritual for Eva and me over the next six weeks.

Our accommodations were adequate, and very clean, although we had to boil our drinking water every morning to be sure of having an adequate supply. We soon became familiar with the routine of leaving the tap on and listening for the water to fill our pour bath with cold water. At 3:00 a.m., I would get up and turn it off. Eva, however, never did become accustomed to taking a cold bath on awakening.

The renovations to the boat were very slow. The dock was twenty-five miles from the compound, and at least once a day we would drive through the heavy traffic to the port where the work was being done. Finally, four weeks after our arrival, the boat was equipped and ready. The staff of the compound, the dentist, Dr. Dorkace Anderson from California, Fred and Polly Ingold, and Rev. Day, as well as Eva and I, accompanied the bishop to the christening of the *Anugra*. While the vessel toured the harbor, the bishop prayed and the men sang Indonesian and English hymns.

All was in order, it seemed, for the vessel to sail at the next high tide. But, as always, there was a hitch. The bishop directed the captain towards the harbormaster's vessel, and he disembarked. After about an hour, he arrived back on the *Anugra*, looking very concerned. He had difficulty in putting on his wide infectious smile. Briefly, he told Dr. Anderson, Eva and myself that there were some very serious problems. He assured us that he was investigating the solution of these serious problems.

Apparently the harbormaster was concerned that there would be missionaries on the vessel who would attempt to convert the residents of the Swamp Islands. The captain told us that the harbormaster had stated that the vessel could not leave port if there were any foreigners aboard.

This problem was never solved. I spent considerable time attempting to get the newly formed Rotary Club to intercede and clear up the confusion, but to no avail. After six weeks in Medan, and much frustration, we departed for home via France.

· Diary of a Miracle ·

After our return from Indonesia in April 1983, we prepared for our next commitment: a visit to India in early September. Once again we would be going at no expense to the project. PDG Dave Kennedy, who is the Rotary CIDA contact in Canada, would be the official representative on behalf of the Canadian committee.

It was now time to write our final report. The most important factors were the study and immunological survey of the red measles immunization project. Dr. Jacob John would spearhead the preparation of this section, and Krish Chitale would be responsible for the overall report, stressing the implementation and organizational aspects of the project.

It had been decided that copies of the report would be sent to Rotary International, CIDA, WHO in Geneva, and UNICEF. The committee sent Dr. Jacob John a letter under the signature of Chairman Paul: It was agreed that the report should include: 1) administration records; 2) documentation of the establishment and maintenance of the cold chain; 3) documentation of the effect on the children. Part 3 would include detailed information about North Arcot District, where 250 children had been immunized, another area, with a further 2,000 population; a rural area with 100,000 population; and a tea estate. All of these areas would be identified by Dr. John.

The report would also include letters and statements of support and approval from prominent government and health officials. It was further agreed that a modest budget of $2,000 would be made available for the Indian committee to cover the costs of serological tests.

Our committee suggested that Dr. Jacob John be appointed chairman, as we expected the report to contain specific acceptable medical surveys. I suggested to the committee that the following Indian Rotarians be involved in their final report: Krish Chitale, C.R. Venkatasubbiah, P.C.M. Sundarapandian, and P.V. Purushothaman.

Eva and I decided to visit Shrinagar before arriving in Madras. We spent four days in this picturesque part of northern India. The scenery was out of this world, resembling the Canadian Rockies, but more primitive. We inspected several houseboats (it is the "in thing" to stay in a houseboat in Shrinagar), but we decided that a small hotel would be more comfortable. Our time there was most enjoyable. The small children of Shrinagar were friendly and polite, and much shyer than the street children of South India, who were always begging for money, or trying to sell us articles of no value.

On our arrival in Madras, Krish was very upbeat about the red measles program. Eva and I looked forward with anticipation to attending a measles camp on the outskirts of Madras. We had worked diligently to achieve this day. The format and infrastructure were simple; Krish and his committee had worked hard and taken everything into consideration. Five nurses—wives of Rotarians—had volunteered to help. They were given instructions regarding the temperature control of the vaccine in large, ice-filled insulated boxes.

They were jovial when we all met at the immunization center, an old office building in one of the poorer districts of Madras. A group of Rotarians were put in charge of handling the children as they arrived with one or both parents. Placed at long tables, their job was to register each child, and give the parents a card of instructions, written in Tamil. Dr. Jacob John had prepared the cards, which alerted parents to possible reactions to the vaccines, explained what reactions were significant and what to do if any reactions occurred.

The Madras Rotary Club had also engaged a town crier, a local resident who toured the immediate vicinity with a drum, calling on the mothers to come out of their huts and take their children to be immunized. For the three previous weeks, local movie theaters had been showing a slide presentation, free of charge, about the measles camp. All we needed now was the children.

Our emotions were up and down like a yo-yo. Would we achieve our target, attracting 3,000 children to be immunized that morning? The medical profession was conspicuous by their absence. However, the two doctors who were present gave a quick course to our volunteers in how to properly place the needle in the outer upper arm area of a child. At first the volunteers were hesitant, but I knew they would soon overcome their fears, and my confidence was not misplaced: they quickly became old pros at the game of immunization.

The two doctors spent most of their time giving brief physical examinations to the children, screening them for any medical problems that would interfere with the action of the vaccine or produce side effects—any serious reactions would, unfortunately, be blamed on the vaccine.

The town crier was very successful. By 9:30, there were long lines of children, in the arms of their mothers, fathers or grandparents, waiting to register. I had the honor of immunizing the first child, who cried, and his mother also shed a tear and thanked me. It was indeed a pleasant reward for all of our previous frustrations.

I remember in particular the camp in Salem. More than 6,000 children were immunized on one very hot, sultry morning. One mother had single-handedly brought her three young children, the eldest of whom was only four. She had carried two, while the four-year-old trudged obediently behind her. When she left the camp, starting across an open field towards her village, I asked Puro to find out how far she had come with her little family. Making inquiries, he discovered that she had walked four and a half miles, and would now walk the same distance home. Women like her were truly the vindication for all the doubts we had encountered and the difficulties we had had to overcome. Eventually, 2.5 million children were immunized by volunteer Rotarians and their wives.

As always, Krish had prearranged our agenda, including trips to Madurai, Trivandrum, Cochin, Calicut, Coimbatore, Salem and Vellore. Dave Kennedy would join us on certain portions of this adventure.

And indeed it was an adventure. Quite apart from any Rotary functions or discussions of the success of the measles program, the train was an experience in itself.

On our way to Trivandrum, we had to make a stopover in a small community where the British had decided to change from a standard-gauge track to a narrow-gauge track when the rail lines were built. Why this was done is known only to God and the engineer who designed the line.

It was 3:30 a.m. when we arrived in this community some seventy-five miles north of Trivandrum, but even at that extraordinarily early hour, we were met and welcomed by a local Rotarian, Dr. Christian, a dentist who lived close by the station. This was not the first time we had been met at this hour of the morning by Rotarians. A year earlier we were met by a Rotarian in Senegal at almost precisely the same hour.

During a Rotary club meeting in Coimbatore, Past District Governor Vadaraj, better known as G.V., presented Eva with a Paul Harris Fellowship. (This is an honor given when one donates $1000 US to The Rotary Foundation; the donor names a recipient for the award. This is one of the methods by which The Rotary Foundation raises money for their activities; at present, they raise over $40 million in US funds each year.)

In his address, G.V. warmly mentioned that Eva was the only woman from Canada who had visited India three times to help with the red measles program. This was three times more than any other Canadian member of the red measles committee. I was proud and honored that she had been recognized. Eva, too, felt flattered and pleased to have been selected to receive this award. It was especially pleasing coming from G.V., who was a warm, sincere man; this was indeed an absolute reward for "service above self."

The praise was particularly welcome as she had previously been unfairly criticized by some volunteer members in their reports. I had also received negative comments on occasion. I would soon learn that the volunteer who was sent with me had included some negative statements about Eva and myself in his report. This did not surprise me: I realized early on in the game that it is easier for some people to criticize rather than be effective.

Perhaps the most memorable adventure was our overnight train trip from Cochin to Madras. The Rotarians had purchased our tickets in Cochin, but unfortunately they could only get accommodations in first class, non-air-conditioned. We were booked in an open compartment with two upper and two lower bunks. The Rotarians had ordered bedrolls for us when we boarded the train.

Shortly after the train left the station, the steward of the coach approached me and asked, "Is there anything you would like, sir?"

"Two bottles of soda," I replied.

"Right, sir," he said, with a royal salute. "At the next station, sir, I will have it."

Ten minutes later, a small man with a self-important-looking cap sat down beside me. "Good afternoon, sir," he said with a broad grin. "I'm your CTI."

In wonderment, I politely asked, "What is a CTI?"

"Well, sir," he said, pointing to the upper part on the compartment, where a line hung from the ceiling. "You see that line? I am the only one on the train who can activate it. If I do, the train stops. Because I am the CTI, better known as the chief ticket inspector." With that he sat down beside me, and asked confidently, "When you boarded the coach, sir, I heard you order three bottles of soda from the steward. Do you have whiskey aboard, sir?"

"No." I replied curtly, hoping to discourage him from further conversation.

Much to my chagrin, he carried on, "The reason I ask, sir, is that like you I enjoy the odd whiskey every now and then, and when I'm the C-T-I it is not illegal."

"I am very sorry, Mr. CTI, but I have absolutely no whiskey with me. I rather enjoy a bottle of Indian soda water."

He stood to take his leave, very much disappointed, I suppose. Before he could get away I quickly asked him where the toilets were on the coach. He told me that this coach had only Asian toilets, and that western toilets were located three coaches ahead. I decided on using the Asian toilet. For those of you who have never had the experience of the Indian railway version of an Asian toilet, I will describe it. It is like our toilets, or an English loo, but without the fixture. It is a plain ten-inch hole in the floor, with foot impressions, directing you where to stand, and a grab rail in front of you. There is another grab rail on the wall behind you, just in case you are squatting. At each station an attendant boards the train and sluices out the toilet by throwing a bucket of Lysol solution on the floor. This does two things; it (supposedly) disinfects the spillage around the hole, and it makes the floor very slippery.

After directing me to the toilets, the CTI departed—only to return like the plague every ten or fifteen minutes to inquire again whether I had any whiskey. Two hours into the trip, and after stopping at several stations, the steward brought in plates of food for the passengers who had ordered their meals at a previous station.

The CTI was soon a permanent fixture at my side. He proceeded to relate his life story, just in case I did have some whiskey to moisten his parched tongue. He had worked on this same run for the past twenty-five years. He also told me that he had overheard my friends ordering bedrolls in Cochin. They would not get them, he said. "Never in those twenty-five years have they ever had bedrolls at the next station."

When we reached the next stop he told us he would now leave us. "I will be turning you over to another CTI," he promised us, " who will look after you till you arrive in Madras tomorrow morning." His parting words still sound in my ears: "Are you sure, sir, that you have no whiskey?" With this he introduced me to his successor and departed our coach.

Back in Madras, Krish had arranged a meeting with Dr. Hande, the state minister of health. The meeting was friendly and sincere. He asked if everything was progressing satisfactorily, and whether the relations between the government and the Rotary committee were cordial. I told him that everything was satisfactory and the project was progressing expeditiously.

He was concerned about what would happen after the last shipment had arrived. This was the opportunity I had been hoping for. It gave me an opening to make two very important points to Dr. Hande. First, I told him that the state must push for the inclusion of measles in the federal government's Expanded Program for Immunization. The inclusion of measles in their EPI would be reviewed in 1985. I related that Dr. Jacob John was most anxious to cooperate with him in order to bring this issue to fruition, not only for the children of Tamil Nadu, but also for all the children of India.

The second matter that I brought to his attention was the urgent need for the state to enter into an agreement to participate in a second-phase measles program, and to guarantee a financial contribution that would increase over a five-year period. With Rotary decreasing its financial support over the same length of time, by 1993 measles immunization would be solely the responsibility of the state.

I told Dr. Hande that this had not been discussed or considered by our committee, but that it was my intention to push for this type of endorsement by his government, our committee, The Rotary Foundation and CIDA. He welcomed the suggestion, and assured me he would explore the possibilities over the next few months. We agreed to meet on my next visit to India.

In Delhi before our return flight to Canada, Rajendra Saboo, the 1981-83 Rotary International director for India (president of Rotary International in 1991-92), invited us to attend the evening social event with the past district governors, present district governors, and the incoming district governors of India. I deemed that Raja was doing me a great honor with this invitation as I had not yet held an office in Rotary. The following day Raja lined up our visit with Dr. Sidhu, the health minister, along with the secretary of the ministry of health.

My discussions with Dr. Sidhu were fruitful. He was planning a trip to Toronto to attend an international health ministers' meeting, and he asked if I would kindly make some arrangements for him concerning Connaught Laboratories. He would be in Toronto on October 8. The meetings I had set up for him had to be cancelled at the last minute, when I received a telephone call from the Indian High Commissioner's office in Ottawa, stating that Dr. Sidhu would unfortunately not be travelling to Canada. I heard later from Raja Saboo, in November, that Dr. Sidhu was assigned an important post in Chandigarh.

In Raja's letter he also stated: "We were so happy to have you at our get-together in Delhi, and indeed to have a person, who has played so significant role as yours in development and implementation of a most exciting 3H program in India, in our gathering was a special privilege for all of us. We enjoyed having Eva and you giving us the benefit of your fellowship and company."

Raja went on to apologize most effusively for my wasted efforts on Dr. Sidhu's behalf.

> I am glad you were able to visit with the health secretary and the minister of health during your stay in Delhi....I deeply appreciate the kind arrangements you made for Dr. Sidhu's visit. Unfortunately, all the arrangements you had made could not be availed of. I do wish to express my gratitude to you for making arrangements in connection with Dr. Sidhu's visit to Canada and organizing to look after him. I owe my apologies also for making you take all the trouble for nothing. On returning to Chandigarh, I talked to Dr. Sidhu and he regrets even more than anyone that he could not have the pleasure of availing the opportunity you had so very kindly and generously laid out for him...you are doing a great work, dear Ken, and we feel proud to belong to an organization which has been enriched by you so much.

Thus the year 1983 ended, on a positive note.

Chapter 23

Early in the New Year of 1984 I received the following telex from Krish: "Received your telex. Vaccine 1.3 million doses in hand. Movie completed editing in progress. Report being circulated among local Rotarians for comments and corrections. Hope you have received draft copy also."

The Canadian red measles committee decided that Chairman Paul and I would go to India in August to wrap up the program. However, in April 1984, I was invited by the incoming president of Rotary International, Dr. Carlos Canseco of Monterrey, Mexico, to be a member of his committee to investigate and explore a proposed project to eliminate polio in the world by the year 2005, the 100th anniversary of Rotary International. This original committee was called "Polio 2005" and later became known as "Polio Plus."

After receiving Dr. Canseco's letter, I replied that I was not a past district governor, nor had I ever been president of our club. His reply was unequivocal and to the point. Briefly, he stated that he wished me to be one of his committee members.

The first meeting was held in Evanston on July 11, 1984, early in the Rotary new year (the Rotary year commences on July 1 each year and ends on June 30 the following year).

Following this three-day meeting, I was asked to visit West Africa to make a preliminary investigation of the reactions of the Rotarians in Cote d'Ivoire, Ghana, Sierra Leone, and Senegal to such a project. President Carlos was planning a visit to this area in the very near future.

This was the first of many personal visits Eva and I would make to Africa.

We arrived in Abidjan, Cote d'Ivoire, at the end of August 1984. Once again I had to rely on my antiquated French in order to communicate. The Rotarians had made appointments with several prominent government officials. Perhaps the Rotarian who influenced me the most was Dr. Constant Roux, a pediatric surgeon. Constant and his wife, Rose, would be dear friends for years. One afternoon, following a tedious, difficult meeting with some government officials, Constant invited us to his home to relax. I remembered him telling me about a small hospital, thirty-five miles east of Abidjan, where he spent ten days a month operating on children who had polio. Suddenly it occurred to me that I would rather make the trip to this center than relax at his home. I asked Constant if he would take Eva and me to visit the hospital; after some persuasion he agreed.

The place was a shock. The emotions I felt on first seeing the children, unable to walk, crawling on their bellies like sand crabs, still haunts me. As I stood with tears in my eyes, I couldn't justify or believe what I was seeing. On my return to Evanston for our meetings in October, I relayed to President Carlos Canseco that he had a 100-percent believer in his proposed program to eliminate polio.

I was also deeply involved in a charitable trust children's hospital in Madras which Krish Chitale had offered to show me one Sunday morning in 1980, when it was just beginning. He was very apologetic, and prefaced his invitation with assurances that it was not his motive to influence me in any manner. As we drove to the center of Madras, Krish described the need for such a non-profit pediatric hospital, which would be available not only to the poorer classes, but also to lower-middle-class workers. We stopped at an older home, painted green.

Entering the house, we were met by a young doctor, who took us to see the patients. There were only four beds, all occupied by very sick infants. Krish explained that 40 percent of the patients were treated free of charge, and the rest paid only minimal amounts for medical treatment.

It was his desire to some day build a first-class hospital for children, which would be the first non-profit charity hospital in South India, as a matter of fact in all of India. That morning I became committed to the cause of the Child Trust Hospital.

Back at home I started to spread the word of this new Madras institution. I was fortunate in getting not only the Rotary Club of Oakville but also the Rotary clubs of Clarkson-Mississauga and North Scarborough to answer my plea for equipment, for this marvelous hospital of mercy. These three clubs responded, and my own Rotary Club responded with a generous donation.

When the board of directors embarked on building a modern facility for the institution, the Rotary Club of Whitby was able to receive a 3H "health, hunger, and humanity" grant from the Rotary foundation for the supply of surgical equipment in the amount of $650,000 (US). This grant was to be supervised by the Rotary Club of Whitby.

It has always astounded me that there was only one other Canadian committee member who helped Krish on this marvelous humanitarian project—Fran Smith, who convinced his club, North Scarborough, to donate some equipment with a matching grant (by which The Rotary Foundation matches the amount budgeted for by a Rotary club for any approved project or program).

In my letter to Krish dated January 31, 1984, I informed him that I had been chosen to be district governor in 1985-86. As we approached the end of the project, I attempted to convince our committee that we must now bring our influence to bear on the Indian governments, at the federal level and at the state level in Tamil Nadu, and convince them that measles must be added to their EPI program. The extension of India's EPI program was to be considered in 1985.

This, to my mind, was crucial. If we genuinely believed that the introduction of red measles vaccine into India was legitimate in the first instance, then we must follow through and make sure that vaccination against measles was included in the government's legislation of 1985. The fact that the treasurer and the chairman were as strongly opposed as

1984

I was in favor was just another minor roadblock, in my view—by this time I was used to negative thinkers, whether they were on the committee or not. I knew that with patience and determination I could overcome the negativism. The question of a second-phase program, in which the state government would contribute on an gradually increasing scale, was also looked on as "impossible." More negativity to overcome.

My letter to Raja Saboo, who later became president of Rotary International (in 1991-92), on January 31, 1984, asked:

> The Canadian measles committee have requested that I write you. We are now in the process of composing our final report, which will be submitted to the 3H Committee of The Rotary Foundation, the Canadian International Development Agency (CIDA), the ministries of health in Tamil Nadu and Kerala, as well as the health officials in New Delhi, UNICEF, WHO, and other interested health agencies in Canada and India.
>
> Our original premise was that when the program was completed, we would be able to convince the health officials in New Delhi that measles should be part of the EPI program, either by importing measles vaccine or by manufacturing it in India....Would we as a Canadian committee be overstepping our mark by approaching either the state or federal ministries of health concerning the inclusion of red measles in India's EPI program? If you personally feel that we would be overstepping our mark, would there be sufficient numbers of interested influential Rotarians who would approach, along with us, the ministries of health and other officials in New Delhi?
>
> A general statement by you to our committee concerning the significance or non-significance of the 3H project, and how it relates to the over-all rural health

care programs, would be much appreciated. Your knowledge, and the respect all Indian Rotarians have for you, indeed places you in a position to be able to answer some of the haunting questions that we are attempting to answer. It is only in answering these questions that we will be able to aid the future generations of Indian children.

In conclusion, I know I have asked you to give some positive answers, and even though your answers may not necessarily be what I wish to hear, it is only through this exchange that you and I as Rotarians are able to offer "service above self." Yours in Rotary, for a better world.

The lack of a negative answer to the above letter consolidated my commitment to future red measles immunization programs in India.

On April 24, 1984, I wrote to Krish:

Our committee in Canada, as well as CIDA and Rotary International, are anxious to bring this project to an historic finish. We must always remember our initial supposition that this project would enable the federal government of India to include measles on its EPI program, either by importing the vaccine or manufacturing the vaccine. It is not enough just to finish the program; but both Indian and Canadian measles committees must make a final concerted effort to make sure that this basic supposition comes to a successful fruition.... Your frustrations, my frustrations, both in the early and latter stages must not be wasted. The two of us must insure that the program is completed and the final report prepared in such a manner that the federal government in New Delhi will encompass our basic premise in their EPI Program, and CIDA as well as Rotary International would consider a red measles immunization program in other districts of India in the future.

Paul McKelvey and I are planning our visit to South India July 15th to August the 4th. You were asking along with the other Rotarians of the Indian measles committee to be sure and bring Eva. As I mentioned the last volunteer in his report stated that she inconvenienced the Rotarians of districts 320 and 321 and tended to be a liability rather than an asset. This will be the first time that my air flight will be covered by the program's budget. I have under obligation accepted this gesture. I will in the near future be forwarding the amount of the air flight to you for deposit into the Child Trust's bank account.

On July 5, 1984, I received a letter from Puro on his arrival in Bombay. Puro and his wife, Jothi, had visited us in Whitby following his training session for incoming district governors in Boca Raton, Florida. He wrote:

I received a telephone call from Paul McKelvey. He informed me of his visit to India from 24th July until 8th August '84. He also told me that you would be in West Africa at that time and would not be able to accompany him. He told me that he had let the Indians know that you would not be coming with him. He knew of the disappointment the Indians would have as well as Krish Chitale and Krishnaswami. Particularly Krish Chitale, who finds a great companion in you.

A further letter from Puro, dated July 14, 1984:

On Saturday the 7th of July the measles immunization committee met at Krish Chitale's....The meeting was a grand success and it was conducted in the presence of Dr. Kapali, Director of Health Services from the state of Tamil Nadu. We are confident of giving the following assurances: The project will be completed by the first week of November '84. Every club has been approached personally and they have been given a target of achieving an immunization of 5,000 children within 3 months' time. This will account for 200,000 doses. I anticipate our district alone will consume 50,000 doses. I am reactivating Dharmapuri District to complete another 50,000 doses.

Meanwhile, our measles program was beginning to get media attention in Canada. *Reader's Digest* was doing a feature article in one of their upcoming editions. I corresponded at the end of July with Mr. Paul Globus and forwarded him a draft copy of the final report.

Chairman Paul's visit to India was very successful. He was able to witness some 11,050 children being immunized in a single day in the Coimbatore area. John Stucky was informed of this accomplishment by telex on August 1, 1984.

Paul's report of his visit was most complimentary to the Indian Rotarians for their ability and continued dedication to this most worthy, altruistic immunization program. In his meeting with the health secretary on August 7, he learned that the state government had recommended that the federal health ministry include measles in their EPI program. He also stated that the government planned to manufacture measles vaccine as soon as possible (however, this has never materialized).

He also asserted that: 1) the Tamil Nadu government will continue to support this program, and with even improved efficiency; 2) the Tamil Nadu government will use its offices to get tax and duty concessions; 3) the Tamil Nadu government will assist Rotary in getting free transport for vaccine, or meet the charges if necessary.

These statements by the state government were indeed refreshing to hear!

In my letter to Krish of November 8, 1984, I made the following estimates of the financial requirements for the continuation of the measles program in Tamil Nadu:

> I estimate that 500,000 doses would be needed yearly. The cost would be $100,000 Canadian dollars. We would expect the state of Tamil Nadu to pick up 20 percent of the cost the first year, or $20,000; the second year 40 percent or $40,000; the third year 60 percent or $60,000; 80 percent the fourth year or $80,000; $100,000 the fifth year and yearly thereafter.
>
> As you know, I am on the Polio Plus committee. At our last meeting I proposed that the state of Tamil Nadu be one of the first Asian areas to participate in this new expanded polio program. President Carlos asked me if I was interested in making early approaches to Dr. Hande. The same conditions would apply if they were approved. Rotary International would supply the oral polio vaccine free of charge for all children under the age of three, for five years. After five years the government would carry on the program. I would appreciate if you would discuss this with Dr. Hande and let me know the result as soon as possible.

The committee asked me to do a final inspection visit in January 1985. This I consented to do, the cost being picked by the project, which in turn I turned over to the Child Trust Hospital, Madras. Eva's airfare was not included. I notified Krish of our planned trip to Madras.

A letter from Puro, dated November 26, 1984, answered the questions I had put to Krish. Yes, Dr. Hande was very interested in the proposed increasing contributions by the state government in a phase-two red measles immunization project. And this response would be returned in writing by the health secretary, within the next two weeks. He also extended an invitation to Eva and me to attend his district conference on January 19-20, 1985, asking me to chair the session on immunization. He kindly ended his letter "Your presence will make the difference for the furtherance of the measles program."

Chapter 24

Our Indian trip to wind up the project was indeed rewarding. I had one unexpected adventure when Raja Saboo asked me to join him in New Delhi and to accompany him when he visited Dr. Bhist, the director general of health services. Mr. K.K. Kapur, the Rotary office manager, accompanied us. Our talks were not especially helpful. Dr. Bhist was a typical bureaucrat. I suggested to Raja that he pursue with the Indian director, Manchandra, the issue of attempting to get an all-India "hold harmless" agreement.

Fortunately, my trip to South India was very productive. I met with Dr. Hande, the minister of health for the state of Tamil Nadu, along with Mr. R. Sanmugan, the secretary of health, and Dr. Kapali, the director of health services, on two occasions. The co-operation that was evident and visible between Rotary and the state government was an example for the rest of the Rotary world to follow. This relationship did not just happen. It had been built up between Dr. Hande, the minister of health, and myself and Krish Chitale over several meetings.

The three of us had a lengthy discussion on the proposed continuation for a second-phase red measles project. However, my concern was to establish a "PANDI" project (PANDI stands for "project of annual national day of immunization") for polio. I was in the early stages of applying, through the Rotary Club of Whitby, for a massive 3H polio-plus immunization program for the state of Tamil Nadu. This would be considered by the programs committee at its June meeting in Las Vegas. Krish, Dr. Hande and I were in full agreement about the necessity of the project for the state of Tamil Nadu. If it was accepted, it would supply oral polio vaccine for all children under the age of three, for a five-year period. A new wrinkle was included on my application. I proposed that $250,000 (US) be included to update the cold chain facilities, i.e., adequate refrigeration units, with standby electrical power sources to provide constant and adequate refrigeration for the vaccine, besides ordinary refrigerators for the storage of vaccine. This was the first Polio Plus project approved that provided for this essential component. I suggested to Dr. Hande that he write a letter to President Carlos Canseco accepting the PANDI philosophy.

He wrote:

> Dear Dr. Carlos Canseco: I have discussed the idea of 'project of annual national day of immunization' (PANDI) approach with Dr. Kenneth Hobbs during his visit to this state of Tamil Nadu. This exciting new approach of polio immunization appeals very much to us. We are hopeful that our state of Tamil Nadu (India), with the population of 48 millions, will be considered as one of the early geographical areas in the world by Rotary International, for this project of polio immunization. The assurance of continuation of the program by our government after five years was stressed by Dr. Hobbs and we are in complete agreement with this philosophy. We eagerly look forward to Rotary International's participation at the earliest.

The above letter was forwarded to President Carlos on my arrival back in Canada. Everything Krish and I had persistently worked for over the past five years was now progressing as we had planned. The satisfactory end of this phase was at hand, and a new adventure was in the making.

· Fall 1984 ·

On March 14, 1985, Governor Puro sent the following telegram to Chairman Paul McKelvey: "Congratulations. Measles project completed. Governor Puroshothaman."

Chapter 25

The meeting of the Canadian committee, on February 12, 1985, dealt with the preparation of our final report and a review of my comments on my most recent trip to India (in January). There was still some resistance from a couple of members of the committee concerning a second-phase program. They felt that our job was finished: we had done what we set out to do.

We discussed the present political uncertainty in the state of Tamil Nadu arising out of the illness of the chief minister, and how it might affect our program. Dr. Hande's position as minister of health could be at risk if a new chief minister was named. Dr. Hande had promised to forward a letter of agreement as soon as his position in the government was clarified, and Dr. Kopali, the director of health services, had assured me that we had nothing to worry about, as he would make sure that the agreement and commitment for a phase-two project would be forthcoming, no matter who was minister of health.

I was very much impressed with Dr. Kopali, and I cannot overemphasize how much I admired Dr. Hande. His honesty and devotion to protecting the health of the children in the state of Tamil Nadu was beyond praise. Over our several meetings we had been drawn into a firm friendship that was based on what we were attempting to do for the health of the children of South India, and on our mutual sense of admiration and respect.

I reported to the committee on my long discussion with health ministry officials on a future "PANDI" polio immunization program.

I had not yet informed the committee that I was planning to submit a 3H application on behalf of the Rotary Club of Whitby for an extensive polio project in the state of Tamil Nadu.

A year later I did submit a 3H application for a $2-million (in US funds) polio project for the state of Tamil Nadu. What made this proposal different was the fact that I applied for $250,000 (US) for a "cold chain" upgrade for the state of Tamil Nadu. After much discussion at the meeting in Las Vegas in late May, the project was endorsed. This was the first Polio Plus project that included a "cold chain" upgrade. An important precedent had been established.

My letter to President Carlos Canseco received a positive reply in a letter to me dated May 28, 1985. He wrote:

> Dear Ken: It gives me great pleasure to inform you that I appoint the following four men to serve with you on 'phase two' of the South India measles project—Paul McKelvey, Wilf Wilkinson, Fred Black and Fran Smith. You may, at your own discretion, add one or two others to this group. Thank you, Ken, for the efforts you are making to discover a new world of service.

The second phase was now up and running. However, there were still a lot of "t"s to cross and "i"s to dot. The first meeting of phase two was called for June 21, 1985. PDG Fran Smith was appointed chairman, as PDG Paul relinquished the chair due to other pressures and responsibilities, PDG Fred Black was appointed secretary, PDG Wilf Wilkinson treasurer and CIDA contact person. My role remained the same, medical consultant for the project.

The application to Rotary International was for $62,800, and to CIDA for the equivalent of $430,800 for a total budget of $493,600 (US). This would supply measles vaccine over the following five years, from 1985 to 1990. The state government was integrally involved, and would contribute 20 percent of the cost of the project in the first year;

40 percent the second year; 60 percent the third year; 80 percent the fourth year and 100 percent the fifth and following years. It was obligatory that Air India transport the vaccine free of charge from New York to Madras. The approval was also conditional upon CIDA's financial involvement.

The conditions in phase two were very different from those of phase one. Merck, Sharpe and Dohme were no longer dispensing the vaccine in multiple-dose vials, and they were not even interested in giving us a quote on a price for multiple-dose vials. The only other large manufacturer of measles vaccine in North America was Connaught Labs of Toronto. They were very interested, as they had already been discussing technology transfer with the government of India for a vaccine-producing plant in Poona, India. However, purchasing from Connaught would mean trucking the vaccine from Toronto to New York. The second major change was that, since the introduction of measles vaccine to the Indian EPI program, all measles vaccine coming into India was required to be tested for potency by the federal government before it could be used. The state of Tamil Nadu then decided that they would do their own potency testing as a precaution. It is interesting to note that since 1979, all through the pilot and initial phases of our measles immunization project, Dr. Jacob John had been potency-testing all of our vaccine.

The real hurdle to jump was the federal government. They were in charge, and this made them responsible for the signing of a new "hold harmless" agreement. These new conditions and changes would result in some long and frustrating lapses of forward movement in our phase two project.

The state government sent their agreement in a letter dated July 4, 1985:

> In continuation of the government letter second cited, I am informed that the government of Tamil Nadu are glad to accept the free offer of measles vaccine made by Rotary International for the next five years with the

financial commitments that the government will fulfill as detailed below:

20 percent of the cost of vaccine in the first year:
    Rs. 2 lakhs [1 lakh equals 100,000]
40 percent of the cost of vaccine in the second year:
    Rs. 4 lakhs
60 percent of the cost of vaccine the third year:
    Rs. 6 lakhs
80 percent of the cost of vaccine in the fourth year:
    Rs. 8 lakhs
100 percent of the cost of the vaccine the fifth year:
    Rs. 10.00 lakhs

Instead of financial commitment on the part of the state government indicated above, the quantity of measles vaccine supplied by the government of India under the expanded immunization programme will be treated as the state's share and, if there is any shortfall, the state government will meet the cost to the extent of the shortfall. R. Shanmugan, IAS, Commissioner and Secretary to Government Health and Family Welfare Department.

This letter was in response to several letters by District Governor Puro of Salem. The commissioner had answered Puro earlier, on June 11, as follows:

Kind attention is invited to your letters cited. I am directed to inform you that the government of Tamil Nadu are glad to accept the offer of measles vaccine made by Rotary International for the next five years. Whatever quantity of vaccine supplied by the government of India will be treated as state's share and if there is any shortfall, the state government will meet the difference in cost. I am also to inform you that the draft agreement in this regard is under scrutiny and will be executed shortly.

Krish forwarded a letter he had received from Dr. Kopali, dated October 4, 1985:

Dear Thiru Chitale: During his address in the central council of health and family welfare, hon'ble minister for health and family welfare, Tamil Nadu, made special mention of the measles immunization program in Tamil Nadu, with the help of Rotary International. The gov't of India has also plans to take more vigorously measles vaccines based on the studies in Tamil Nadu. We have addressed government of India regarding their concurrence for hold harmless agreement. Soon after its receipt I will contact you. Dr. V. Kopali.

As a member of The Rotary Foundation's 3H committee, I attended my first meeting in October 1985. The 3H grant for the phase-two measles program was approved. A second project in which I was principally involved was also approved. I had convinced our district to become involved in a workshop for rehabilitation of the handicapped, in co-operation with the Rotary Club of Madras and "WORTH" (WORTH stands for "workshop for the handicapped"—this was started by the Swiss Red Cross several years ago; it is a non-profit enterprise). I had first seen the WORTH workshop in Vellore in 1980.

I was so impressed with their program for rehabilitating handicapped persons that I pursued the idea of our district implementing such a project with district funds, CIDA funds and Rotary International 3H funds. Our World Community Service District Committee collected $75,000 from the clubs in our district, The Rotary Foundation contributed

$100,000, and CIDA contributed $340,000, for a total budget of $510,000. This would provide a workshop of trained personnel to supervise and train twenty handicapped students a year.

Most of these handicapped persons would be females. There is only one thing worse than being handicapped in the developing world, and that is being female and handicapped in the developing world. This project would train handicapped persons to become electronic technicians, thus affording them an open door to be self-supporting. This project was also passed by the Rotary International 3H committee in October 1985.

My dream that measles would be included in India's expanded program of immunization had become a reality. On November 25, 1985, I opened a letter from Governor Puro, and read:

> Yesterday evening when I tuned up to listen to the television news which is broadcast throughout India, I listened to a special bulletin and the points of interest are as follows: 1) measles have been included in the 'universal immunization program.' 2) Government of India will receive 64,000,000 doses of measles vaccine for immunizing the entire children in Andrah Pradesh, as well as the tribal areas. The man behind the entire success of the measles immunization program is nobody else than Ken Hobbs. I would request you to kindly share this information with your team members! P. V. Puroshothaman.

Chapter 26

The first committee meeting of 1986 was held on the 9th of January. The committee members were apprehensive. This was the first time they had been subjected to the frustrating indecisiveness, or even complete refusal to make decisions, of the federal and state governments of India. The required approvals had not as yet been granted. Locally, we were still waiting for a firm quote on the price of the vaccine from Connaught Laboratories. CIDA had not committed itself to financial support for phase two of our red measles immunization project.

After nine months of intensive planning, we still had not advanced one step toward activating phase two. The committee met again in early February, while Krish Chitale was in Canada to attend my district conference as a speaker on our district's WORTH project in Madras. At this meeting, before he returned to India, Krish expressed the view that the fall of 1988 would be the earliest that the project could be implemented.

Connaught Labs finally issued a quote of 17 cents per dose for the Schwartz strain of measles vaccine, rather than the Edmonston strain which had been used in the pilot and phase one. At the end of March 1986 the following telex was sent to Krish Chitale: "CIDA has approved measles 'phase two.' Please inform when Air India has granted free shipment. Ken."

Krish advised me that Dr. Hande had received a letter from the minister of health and family welfare in New Delhi concerning the federal government's ability to supply the state of Tamil Nadu's agreed-upon share of doses. They requested that they be given an adequate advance warning. He also forwarded a long, confusing legal statement regarding the minister's responsibility in the matter of signing a "hold harmless" agreement with Rotary International. This was written by R.N. Poddar, a solicitor for the ministry.

During my year as governor, I had planned a family exchange trip to India and South India, lasting from February 20 to March 21, 1986. Eleven couples, including Eva and myself, toured the highlights of North India and South India. The trip was a very enjoyable and illuminating experience for all group members.

It also afforded me the opportunity of attending a meeting with Dr. Hande and the district governors of Districts 320, 321, 322, 323. The meeting was also attended by the new director of the government's pediatric hospital. He expressed concern that phase two had not been implemented, with the result that there had been a huge outbreak of measles in South India; in the Madras area it was an epidemic.

During my meeting with the Canadian High Commissioner in New Delhi, he insisted that I must pursue the funding issue in Ottawa with CIDA immediately on my return. He agreed to inform CIDA of his personal concern over the delay in granting funding to phase two.

Before going to India in February, I had been invited by Connaught Labs to attend a reception in Ottawa on January 22, 1986. They were celebrating a successful technology transfer: the establishment of a vaccine production unit in Pakistan. At this reception I met Mr. Alun Davies, the president of Connaught Labs, as well as Mrs. Margaret Catley-Carlson, the president of CIDA. I also had a lengthy discussion with Mr. Gilles Cossette, the vice-president in charge of marketing for Connaught Labs. On my return from India I had lunch with Mr. Cossette. We discussed Connaught Laboratories' interest in a technology transfer project with India for the production of trivalent oral polio, measles and other vaccines. He expressed interest in a combined approach to Ottawa with our committee. He also suggested that our committee should tour Connaught Labs at the end of April. This visit took place, and we began discussions about the possibilities of technological transfer.

· Diary of a Miracle ·

On March 27, 1986, CIDA gave its approval for financial contributions of $218,500 for phase two. The project's authorized budget was as follows:

Expenditures:

3.0 million doses of measles vaccine
at 20 cents per dose ....$ 600,000.00
Canadian administration ....$ 17,000.00
Total $617,000.00

Income:

Rotary clubs in India
Air India
State governments and others ....$ 320,000.00
Rotary district 707:
Project $70,000.00
Administration $8,500.00
Total $78,500.00

CIDA:
Project $210,000.00
Administration $8,500.00

Total ....$ 617,000.00

CIDA's grant of $ 218,500 would be spread over five years as follows:

First year ....$ 61,700.00
Second year ....$ 61,700.00
Third year ....$ 47,700.00

Fourth year ....$ 31,700.00
Fifth year ....$ 16,700.00
Total ....$ 218,500.00

Dr. Jacob John forwarded a copy of a letter, which he had received from the honorable minister of health, the significant part of which read:

> ...however, for procuring vaccines from the Rotary International for the current year, i.e. 1985-86, we have no objection provided the state gov't satisfies itself about quality of vaccine supplied and makes adequate arrangements to test specifications before use or that arrangements be made so that Rotary International will inform the state government about sources of procurement and the purchase of vaccines will be made from such manufacturers who comply with the WHO requirements relating to specifications, testing, quality control, etc.

"Based on this letter," Dr. Jacob John wrote, "we might be able to get customs duty clearance."

For a while, there was no significant activity in phase two. During the lull, I made an application for a Polio Plus grant for the state of Tamil Nadu, in the name of the Rotary Club of Whitby, in the amount of $2.5 million (US). This application included $250,000 for the cold-chain upgrade. I also suggested to Past President Carlos Canseco that we invite Mr. Alun Davies from Connaught Labs to address The Rotary Foundation's programs committee at our meeting in Las Vegas in early June 1986. This was accomplished. Mr. Alun Davies addressed the committee, and suggested that Rotary International and Connaught Labs jointly pursue the establishment of a technological transfer of vaccine production with the government of India. Unfortunately this was never followed up successfully. My Polio Plus project was approved for the state of Tamil Nadu, including the $250,000 (US) for cold-chain upgrading.

Herb Pigman, the secretary general of Rotary International, would be in New Delhi and Madras in early August 1986, to consummate the Polio Plus agreement with the Rotarians and the local state government of Tamil Nadu. Krish extended an invitation for me to attend, as did District Governor Ramakrishnan.

At our committee meeting on July 29, it was decided that Chairman PDG Fran Smith would be the first volunteer for phase two. His visit would be in mid-September. The first shipment of vaccine was scheduled for September 24, 1986. I also informed the committee that Dr. Hande would no longer be the health minister, due to his recent electoral defeat. The logistics of shipping the vaccine from Toronto to New York and then on to Madras were worked out. The committee hoped that Connaught Labs would follow and approve the format. They accepted our suggestions.

On September 6, 1986, I received the following telex from Krish: "Approvals not obtained from Delhi. Request postponement Fran's visit. Will telex you once approval obtained." Two days later, there was another telex: "Please advise number of doses and origin of vaccine and port of loading."

Perhaps the only real positive action for me in 1986 was being asked by John Stucky of Rotary International to visit Georgetown, Guyana, in September. The Singer sewing machine company had abandoned their manufacturing plant in Guyana a few years earlier, and they were having difficulty getting their last bank account cleared by the government. They decided to give the money to Rotary and other charities; $100,000 was earmarked for Rotary International, providing Rotary could design a project or projects which would benefit the local people.

John Stucky asked me to go to Georgetown for a week to ten days, during which time I would work in co-operation with, and advise, the local Rotary Club in designing a project or projects that would be acceptable to The Rotary Foundation. I left Toronto on August 25 and returned on September 6.

In Georgetown, local Rotarians and I together looked at several suggestions from club members. Finally, on my last day, we came up with two worthwhile projects.

The first one was to design and equip a trailer that could travel up and down the coast, checking and recording the status of each and every child as to age, weight, height, vision, and hearing ability. Almost 80 percent of the population of Guyana lives within five miles of the seacoast. The results of this survey would be ongoing. The project would yield a reliable report on the health and nutrition of the children of Guyana.

The second project was designed to offer aid to handicapped persons. A chick hatchery would be set up. Each handicapped person in the country would be given a certain number of chicks, and an appropriate amount of feed, yearly. The project would last five years, after which time it would be self-supporting as a co-operative. This would give the handicapped, who were considered a financial drain on the country, a chance to establish some independence. The handicapped persons would earn their own money and make their own decisions, for example, as to whether they would market the eggs or raise the chicks for food. These two projects were approved by the 3H committee in October 1986.

Two years later, in April 1988, when I once again visited Guyana on a Polio Plus survey, I was privileged to attend the official opening of the chick hatchery project!

The year ended with no government approvals and no plans for a first shipment of vaccine in phase two. All of our plans seemed to be up in the air. The members of our committee were in a quandary. How were they to proceed?

As for me, I have never forgotten what Krish told me in 1979: "This is India, Ken. You must have patience." And patience I have always had, since that remarkable day in 1979—at least as far as India is concerned.

Chapter 27

In mid-January 1987, Connaught Labs invoiced the committee for measles vaccine that was being held by them in storage. Chairman Fran Smith sent a letter to each committee member on January 26, stating that the treasurer reported that Connaught Labs wanted to know whether we were willing to release the vaccine that we had in storage so they could utilize it elsewhere. The committee decided to reject this request. We were all optimistic that our Indian government agreement problems would be solved in the immediate future.

The chairman was becoming very anxious, and in his frustration sent the following telegram to Krish Chitale on January 29, 1987: "Regret to advise unless we receive clearance to ship measles vaccine held in long overdue storage by February 15th, we must release to Connaught in order to receive repayment at full value. Any continued delay might precipitate withdrawal from project which would be tragic. Please convey our position to appropriate decision making authority. Reply by return wire is essential. Fran Smith."

Ten days later, on February 8, the following reply was received by telex: "Ref to Fran Smith telegram. C.T. and I visited Delhi seventh to push approvals. Request Fran Smith and members to give us time till fifteenth March to sort out problems. We are still interested in implementing program. We are equally concerned about approvals. Many happy returns to Eva. Krish."

On February 27, 1987, Mr. P.K. Umashankar, the national Secretary of Health and Family Welfare, wrote to Shri R. Shunmugham, his counterpart in the government of Tamil Nadu, as follows:

> Kindly refer to your letter No. 83539aA/P2/86-1, dated 2-12-1986, to the Director General of Health Services, relating to importing 1.5 million doses of measles vaccine by the Rotary International (District 707 Canada). You have sought clearance of the Government of India under the Drug Control Act and also permission for import of the vaccine into India. I am enclosing herewith a copy of notification issued by the Department of Revenue in the Ministry of Finance indicating that measles vaccine is exempted from import duty, subject, however, to the execution of a bond. Hence, I presume you do not require any import clearance by DGHS. I may add that we have no objection to your importing this vaccine for use in connection with the immunization programme sponsored by the state government.
>
> Customs Declaration No. 3892/86 dated 13-7-1986: G.S.R. 950(e) in exercise of the powers conferred by subsection (1) of section 25 of the customs act, 1962 (52 of 1962), the central government being satisfied that it is necessary in the public interest so to do, hereby makes the following further amendment in the notification of the Government of India in the Ministry of Finance (Department of Revenue) No. 45-Customs, dated the 1st March 1979, namely…[*It goes on for another page and in conclusion it will include measles vaccine to be admitted free of customs duty.*] With regards, P.K. Umashankar.

The way was now cleared, after months of haggling and frustration, for our committee and the Indian committee to proceed with phase two.

Along with the measles vaccine dilemma, I had been working on the new 3H project, specifically, the rehabilitation workshop. This had been approved conditionally by the 3H committee, if CIDA funding was approved. PDG Dave Kennedy, who was the Rotary-CIDA go-between, turned down CIDA's participation in our proposed project, because (as he stated on more than one occasion) "handicapped people are not cost-effective." After CIDA had turned down the financing, I had to persuade the 3H program to allow us to go ahead with the project without CIDA funding. They gave their decision in the following telex to me: "The following telex sent today to Rotarian K.V. Shetty, Rotary Club of Madras: 'Pleased to inform you that the trustees have approved the waiver of CIDA funding contingency. Amount of 3H grant remains unchanged at US $93,000. We are processing initial payment of US $44,000. All necessary documents are now on file.' Best wishes, Terri Hennes, 3H Grants Coordinator."

Rotarian Bill Nurse and his wife Mae were the first volunteers for the WORTH project. Needless to say, their contribution of time and effort was made at no cost to the project. They arrived in Madras in late March. To demonstrate what a generous and worthwhile Rotarian he is, at the opening ceremony of the WORTH project, Bill handed over his own personal check for $100,000 because the money had not arrived from our district and Rotary International.

Phase two was now in high gear with the receipt of the following telex from Krish on April 13th: "Free transportation thru Air India arranged. Send shipment dates. Regards, Chitale."

I sent the following telex to Krish on May 6, 1987:

> Measles vaccine departs JFK New York 20:15 May 11 Flt 102. Arrives Bombay 0200 May 13. Connects AI flt 402 May 13 0600. Arrives Madras 0750 May 13. Imperative that this connection is made in Bombay as ice time for vaccine is critical otherwise vaccine must be in cold storage. Please insure that the connections are

1987

made between flights in Bombay on May 13. Fran Smith arrives in Madras on May 14th. Telex to follow. Please acknowledge this telex immediately, by return telex. Ken Hobbs.

On May 13, the following telex was received:

400,000 doses of measles vaccine arrived this morning and stored at King Institute. Please inform concerned people. Received WORTH. Also Bill's WORTH parcel. Shall reply in due course. Krish Chitale.

Chairman Fran Smith arrived in Madras on May 14 and departed on May 29. Fran visited Tiruchirapalli (better known as Trichi), Madurai, Coimbatore, Salem, Vellore, and Madras. He was very surprised at the continuance of the interest and enthusiasm for measles vaccination, when they were now entering a massive five-year polio project concurrently. The program was on full throttle.

In mid-July I received a phone call from John Stucky of the 3H program, asking if I would volunteer to join a group to visit Africa on a Polio Plus exploratory program. I would be joining a staff member, as well as Dr. Hector Acuna from Mexico, a past director of PAHO (Pan-American Health Organization). Hector was a dear friend. He also had served on the Polio 2005 committee with me in 1984-85. He was also a consultant to the Programs Committee of The Rotary Foundation.

We were to meet in Abidjan on September 1. From there we would visit Guinea, Conakry; Lome, Togo; Doualla, Yaounde, Cameroon; Kinshasa, Zaire; Brazzaville, Congo; Nairobi, Kenya; Antananarivo, Madagascar; and Kigali, Rwanda. Our mission was to discuss "mass polio campaigns" with the Rotarians in each country, UNICEF and health ministry officials. I arrived home on October 2.

While visiting a government hospital in Doualla, Cameroon, I was shocked. While touring this facility I happened to notice a small structure on the outer perimeter of the hospital. It was approximately 25 feet by 25, painted white, and appeared to be new.

"What is that?" I asked one of the Rotarians who was accompanying Dr. Hector and myself.

"That's our blood lab. Would you like to see it?"

"Certainly," I answered.

As we got closer to the building I could clearly see the "Rotary wheel." (This was the early symbol of Rotary. It represented the fact that the meetings rotated from place to place. It was finally adopted as our official symbol in 1912. It has twenty-six cogs and eight spokes and a keyway in the middle of the hub, which allows the wheel to be a worker rather than an idler.) The Rotarian who was escorting me went on to tell me that Rotary clubs in the Netherlands and Sweden had established this facility as the first blood transfusion center in Cameroon. The building was meticulous inside and out. It was extremely clean and bright. The blood letting room was impeccable, and the storage facilities for typed and tested blood were unbelievably clean by African standards.

However, as I talked with the technician, I realized that, according to what I was being told, the blood was not typed or cross-matched before being given as a transfusion to a patient, and that this is the normal practice in most of new independent African states, because their finances do not permit such an extravaganza of basic scientific procedures, although the medical community has, over the years since the Second World War, accepted that these are of paramount importance. He further related to me that approximately 45 percent of the blood tested was rejected, because of AIDS, syphilis or hepatitis B.

Ever since that day I have been upset. Every morning while shaving I tell myself again that this is a tragedy that ought to be prevented. The typing and cross-matching of blood is not a new discovery. It has been implemented in most of the world since the early 1930s. The question I ask myself is always the same: What am I willing to do to correct the situation?

I vowed that this great injustice and inequality would be corrected.

I have attempted to correct this intolerable situation by applying to Rotary International for a $300,000 3H grant, conditional upon CIDA giving another $2-million grant (in US funds). The project would provide for the establishment of a national blood transfusion service in Cote d'Ivoire, Ghana, Sierra Leone, Burkina Faso and Mali. The project would equip laboratories in these five countries, train technicians for five months on how to type, cross-match, and test blood for AIDS, syphilis and hepatitis B. In addition, a nurse would be trained to aseptically collect and administer blood for transfusions. A medical doctor would become the chief of the blood transfusion service after his or her training. The committee of the Rotary Club of Whitby decided that this training would be in Monterrey, Mexico, where there were bilingual French technicians, and where The Rotary Foundation had invested a large sum of money to provide for the production of inexpensive blood reagents for typing and cross-matching blood. We also recognized that such trainees would be better prepared for the differences in their social environment than if they were trained in the United States or Canada.

After a visit to Geneva, visiting WHO and the International Red Cross, to enlist aid and endorsement, and two special visits to these countries in 1988 and 1989, all at considerable personal expense, we were finally prepared to present our case to CIDA in Ottawa.

We were quickly turned down by CIDA.

Even though they had been thoroughly briefed during our committee's investigative process, they preferred to give $10 million (Cdn) for a government-to-government program to produce a comic book to teach young teenagers of some Southern African countries about the dangers of unsafe sex, and how to properly use a condom. In their wisdom, they apparently thought that was a better investment for Canadian taxpayers than setting up a national blood transfusion center in each of these five countries.

The new regulations concerning potency testing of the vaccine were now in force. The vaccine that arrived on May 13 was stored in the King Institute until August. Finally, the government of Tamil Nadu sent samples to Kasauli, which is near Chandigarh in North India. All of this delay and inefficiency was the responsibility of the assistant drug controller in New Delhi, who had issued a proclamation that all vaccines must be potency-tested before they would be released. In September, four months after their arrival, the tests were finished at last, and the vaccine was ready to be administered.

    The year 1987 ended on a positive note. Phase two was in go-ahead mode.

Chapter 28

While I was in Africa in the fall of 1987, President Chuck Keller asked me to be his personal representative at district conferences scheduled for January 1988 for Districts 310 and 320 in India. This would give me an opportunity to visit Madras and explore the activities of phase two.

Our treasurer had been in touch with CIDA on January 5, 1988, through our Rotary contact, PDG Dave Kennedy, explaining the reasons for the apparent delay in implementing phase two. The government's breakdown, after the apparent assassination attempt on Prime Minister Rajiv Gandhi, had prevented the first shipment of vaccine, which was due to be sent in December 1985. Then, the import permit and the "hold harmless" agreement were not received till March 1987, and the first shipment of 400,000 doses arrived in May 1987. A further reason was a new Indian government policy that required testing the vaccine for potency; there were many delays and the results of these tests were not made available till October 1987. After this date, the vaccine shipped in May could be used. PDG Kennedy informed CIDA that, with luck, we would be able to ship another 400,000 doses in March of this year.

Dr. Jacob John released his tests, requested by the state of Tamil Nadu, on the potency of the vaccine to Dr. N.C. Appavoo, deputy director of public health and preventive medicine (immunization) on January 4, 1988. The results, signed by Dr. Vinohar Balraj, were as follows:

· Diary of a Miracle ·

Batch No.	Expiry date	Titter (T50/0.5mml)
1) 4305-11	5/88	Less than 10
2) 4306-11	6/88	Less than 10
3) 4308-11	6/88	Less than 10
4) 4309-11	6/88	Less than 150
5) 4305-11	6/87	Less than 10 (received by us on 18/11/87)

Titters with values of 10 and above are considered to be within the satisfactory range

10^3 TCID 50 equals 1000 TCID 50.

The above potency testing showed that we had a problem with the vaccine sent in May 1987.

When I visited the King Institute in Madras on January 21, I was alarmed to find some distinct changes in the color-coding that indicated the stability of the temperature environment of the vaccines. I thoroughly checked the recorded information concerning the temperature readings of their walk-in freezer lockers since the arrival of the vaccine in May '87. The records were absolutely positive for the fact that the temperature had not varied inthat time. I then sent the following telex to Mr. Alun Davies of Connaught Labs:

> Re Rotary measles program. Color indicators are in B to C category, expiry date May-June 1988. Has been kept at 2 to 8 degrees C. Potency levels dropping. Is it possible to store vaccine at minus 20 deg C to preserve potency. Urgent reply requested.

I received the following reply from Robert Sloan of Connaught Labs on February 1, 1988:

> Re Rotary measles category—your telex to Mr. Davies: Our regulatory affairs department advises that product should remain in storage at 2 to 8 degrees C until more information is obtained.
>
> 1) Please advise us of potency levels you have determined.
> 2) Have cold chain monitors shown movement to b and c categories recently or during transit to India?
> 3) Please send 10 vials vaccine and diluent for testing. Product should be sent in insulated cartons with ice packs to ensure refrigerated temperatures maintained.

Before returning home I was asked to be guest speaker at the Rotary Club of Madras. Susheila (Krish's wife) had recently suffered a myocardial infarction. We had decided years ago that, in honor of all the care, attention and hospitality that she extended to every volunteer on this and all previous measles programs since the very beginning in 1979, we would make her a Paul Harris Fellow, and now we put our intentions into effect.

A write-up in the Madras Club's *Bulletin* of January 26, 1988, reads:

> Among other things Rotarian PDG Ken Hobbs touched upon the overwhelming hospitality extended to his wife Eva and to him during his seven trips to India. As a measure of the great understanding and good will of this great nation and the tremendous services rendered by the Rotarians of Tamil Nadu in general and in particular the yeoman services rendered by Rotarian PHF PP. S.L. Chitale to the measles/polio programme, he announced,

amidst thunderous applause, that Eva and himself have much pleasure to nominate RTN Ann Susheila Chitale as a Paul Harris Fellow. This is a great gesture on the part of Dr. Hobbs, demonstrating the Rotarian International motto 'Service above Self.'

We record our deep appreciation and gratitude to Rotarian PDG Dr. Ken Hobbs—a dedicated Rotarian—one in a million—and wish that his traits grow in abundance. There has been a saying that behind the success of any man, there is a woman. We are aware that Ann Susheila has spared Rotarian PP S.L. Chitale to give full-time service to Rotary. She richly deserves our admiration. We congratulate her on becoming a Paul Harris Fellow.

On my return home I contacted Connaught Labs. They assured me that they had re-tested samples from their own file. These proved to be potent and showed no signs of deterioration. I had suggested that they place the temperature monitoring devices in direct contact with the vials. They accepted this as a good idea and agreed to pursue this approach.

Dr. Jacob John wrote Connaught Labs on my advice on March 16, 1988. In his letter, he states:

> We had repeatedly tested the four samples in vero cells and found the vaccine titter to be less than ten. Since Connaught vaccine is prepared in chick embryo cells (CEF) we also tested the four batches in CEF cells. Again the titters were undetectable…In February we inoculated five monkeys with 0.5 ml of vaccine batch No. 4308-11. All monkeys developed HAI antibody titters of 16(1), 32(2), 128 (2). Thus the vaccine has sufficient residual potency to immunize monkeys. The vaccine has been kept between 4 and 8 degrees C.

Dr. Webber, directory of regulatory affairs of Connaught Labs, wrote to Jacob John on March 22, 1988. "I am not certain what further steps are required to obtain full clarification of the potency matter. Please be assured that we will do what we can to assist you in this."

Eva and I left Toronto on April 21 for two investigative trips for the 3H committee. the first destination was Georgetown, Guyana, where I had volunteered in September 1986. This time it would be to scrutinize Guyana's Polio Plus program. I had the opportunity to also explore the two 3H programs I had helped to establish in 1986. After we finished our four days in Georgetown, we headed for Bogota, Colombia, to execute a site visit on a proposed 3H project. It would provide a play area and nutritional feeding center in a slum area outside of Bogota.

Back in Madras, the mystery of lost potency continued. The Child Trust Hospital sent a member of their staff to our hospital in Whitby for a six-week orientation period. Meena was asked to bring with her refrigerated samples of vaccine from the May 1987 shipment, which she agreed to do. The vaccine arrived in Whitby with Meena on May 2 and was transferred immediately to Connaught Labs for testing. On May 19, I learned from Connaught Labs that the potency testing on the samples from India showed that they were potent, and had not deteriorated.

I immediately phoned Jacob John in Vellore. After a long conversation we concluded that it could only be his cell culture in Vellore that was at fault and this was the reason that the tests showed no potency. He assured me that he would change the cell culture immediately. Another unpleasant problem was now solved, which had once again delayed our phase two project.

After informing Krish of the solution of our potency problems, he suggested that the second shipment of phase two be in January 1989.

The staff of the 3H program asked me to do a final site inspection in early September 1988 in West Africa; it was one of the first 3H projects, a hospital some 500 miles east of Bamako, Mali, on the fringe of the Sahara Desert in a place called Sen, which is some seventy-five miles from Tombouctou. The project had been designed by a French district; my assignment, along with another doctor, was to inspect the hospital facilities.

Eva and I arrived in Bamako and joined up with our companions, a French non-Rotarian doctor who had worked on several occasions in the hospital and came to Sen at his own expense, and the president of the Rotary Club of Bamako. During my cursory reading of the material sent to me from Rotarian International by the 3H staff, I had noted that the living conditions in Sen were appalling. I suggested to Eva that we should pack sheets with our clothing. She disagreed, pointing out that sheets would surely be available at our destination. However, without telling her, I did pack two sheets.

Our trip from Bamako to Sen was long, hot and dusty. We departed Bamako at 10:00 a.m. and finally entered Sen, which was south of Tombouctou, at 11:00 p.m. We first went to the falling-down old town hall, but there was nobody around. The president of the Bamako club drove us to a local Rotarian's home. The French flew fast and furious. I was only able to pick up the odd word. Eva kept asking, "What are they saying?" I tried to satisfy her that all was well.

Finally, at midnight, we left the Rotarian's home and returned to the town hall, where I was told we would be staying in the town hall guest room.

We climbed the dark stairway to the third floor, becoming more suspicious with each step we took that we were in for a horrendous experience. Eva dug out the tiny flashlight she always carries in her purse. The four of us were now on the third floor of the old town hall, and two things were obvious: that there were two bedrooms and two bathrooms, and that the plumbing had not been working for several years. The odor was execrable.

On entering the master suite we were welcomed by a bed which was covered with bird droppings. The mattress was stained from one end to the other. No sheets or towels were evident.

Eva exclaimed in frustration, "Why did you listen to me about the sheets?"

"I didn't," I replied. With that I looked for the cleanest place on the floor to open my suitcase. When I pulled out two sheets she almost cried for joy.

The night was long and cool. There was no window glass. Two crows kept passing through our room most of the night. The morning presented new opportunities for excitement. How does one wash, shave and toilet, when there is only a trickle of water? The washbasin, toilet, and bidet were dirty, cracked and odoriferous. While attempting to brush my teeth with a small bottle of water (which we have learned always to carry) I could hear the conversation across the hall.

The French doctor was saying that he would not stay another night in these accommodations. The president of the Bamako club understood and agreed. They said in French that they would tell Eva and me at breakfast that they felt these accommodations were not suitable for Eva.

We had breakfast at a small restaurant on the outskirts of the town. During breakfast a storm of dust suddenly blew up; it was a Mazda Land Rover, out of which emerged several smiling people, including a very jovial individual, who came and sat at our table. He introduced himself as the president of the Chamber of Commerce of Tombouctou. He invited us to visit his city, which was only seventy-five miles away. We unfortunately had to decline his kind invitation.

After his departure the Bamako club president brought up the problem of the accommodations. I attempted to relieve his concern, but to no avail. He said that he would take us to visit the local military commandant at the fort.

From his conversations in French with the commandant, I gathered that he was asking permission for us to stay at the summer retreat of the president of Mali. This was a place used only occasionally by the president. I sensed another experience in the making.

The hospital we came to see was worth all the difficulties we had had to put up with. Two operating theaters had been re-equipped with up-to-date surgical tables, operating room lights, and surgical equipment with above average sterilizing facilities. As I walked around the facility, it once again made me proud to be a Rotarian.

The president's retreat was another experience that we will always remember. Our bedroom belonged to the president. It had a king-sized bed with a decorated headboard of mirrors. Mirrors, mirrors, everywhere. The sheets were obviously not clean, so once again our sheets came out of the suitcase. Our sleep was at least uninterrupted.

After breakfast we started the long trip back to Bamako.

I had also been asked to visit Burkina Faso and inspect an earthen dam project. This in itself was another remarkable project, built with a 3H grant of $200,000 (US), some twenty-five miles outside of Ouagadougou.

The dam was approximately three hundred feet in width, with cement spillways that had been constructed on a small stream. After two monsoon seasons, they now had a lake thirty-five by fifteen kilometers in area, and thirty-five meters deep at its deepest point. Farmers had built their homes all around the lake. When we took our leave, the chief of the village presented Eva and me with a live chicken as a gift, in honor of what Rotary International had accomplished for these impoverished farmers.

We also visited Mauritania to get an update on a potential Polio Plus project. Our Rotarian guide, a dentist, gave us a complete tour of all the rehabilitation facilities.

Perhaps the most fascinating part of our trip from a historical point of view was a visit to Guinea Bissau. Rotary was attempting to start a club here, sponsored by the main Dakar, Senegal, club. I did some preliminary work and inquired about the almost nonexistent health care system in this old Portuguese colony. The poverty was indescribable. There were no local or imported newspapers because there was no paper. There were no radio or TV stations, because all electricity was produced by gasoline generators. This colony was an entity unto itself. The only hotel was called September the 25th, after their revolution and separation from the rest of Africa. The way into and out of Guinea Bissau was by a DC3 on Mondays, Wednesdays and Fridays, from Banjul in the

Gambia. Our departure was delayed because of the closing of the airport in Banjul. I was told at the Quonset-hut air terminal, by a very interesting young man who spoke faultless English, that the Americans were sending up a spaceship, and that the airport in Banjul would be closed until 7:00 p.m. because it had been designated the first emergency retrieval station in this space flight.

On our arrival home I received a request to do a site visit to Monterrey, Mexico, to explore another potential 3H project; this one was a hearing loss prevention program. This trip would also allow us to attend Past President Carlos and Maria Canseco's youngest son's wedding. There is nothing more magnificent than a formal Mexican wedding.

In mid-November, an order was placed with Connaught Labs for 400,000 doses of measles vaccine, for delivery to India in mid-January 1989.

Chapter 29

*O*nce again the treasurer appeared to have appointed himself chairman and committee of one, without consulting the other committee members, wrote Dave Kennedy, the coordinator for Rotary CIDA funds. He explained that we had ongoing difficulties in maintaining the immunization schedule in this phase of the project. The committee refused to ship any further vaccine until the shipment of May 1987 had been totally distributed.

The treasurer wrote, "We have recently been advised by the Indian government that they are now in a position to continue the project. We have ordered a second shipment from Connaught Labs, which will be sent shortly. We hope to receive Air India's guarantee of free shipment momentarily. The committee has only met twice in the past year. However, Dr. Ken Hobbs has been on top of the situation with frequent telephone calls to Krish Chitale in Madras."

Shortly thereafter, I received a copy of a letter from Krish, which was written to him by Dr. Dorijan, the director of public health, in which he states:

> The Rotary international supplied 4.00 lakhs [4.00 lakhs equals 400,000 doses] of measles vaccine during the year 1987-1988, and all of these vaccines were utilized fully, by immunizing the children against measles, throughout the state along with the government of India's supplied vaccines.

During the year 1988-89 6.44 lakhs [640,000] children up until October 1988 were immunized against measles as per agreement of government of Tamil Nadu. The share part of the government by means of vaccine supply has been fully met with.

We are agreeable to the Rotary import of 1,00,000 doses of measles vaccine during January 1989 which can be absorbed by the state.

Dr. Dorijan also outlined their strategy for measles immunization:

Immunization programs are being organized on all Wednesdays in rural areas of Tamil Nadu, and in urban areas it is being done on all Saturdays, for outreach immunization activities. The program is being carried out in 12,616 village panchayats, 98 municipal panchayats, 8 townships, 2 cantonments, 98 municipalities, and in 3 corporations. Immunization services are also provided daily at hospitals like District Headquarters hospitals (19), Taluk hospitals (125), non-Taluk hospitals (120), ESI Hospitals, and dispensaries (139), in addition to private nursing homes and clinics. As such it is laborious procedure to furnish clinic-wise data on measles immunization. However, the beneficiaries in each year from 1987 to1989, and the vaccine supply are furnished below.

The measles immunization achievement was as follows:

Year	Target in lakhs	Achievement in lakhs
1987-88	6.77	10.79*
1988-89	8.73	10.67
1989-90 (up to Dec. 89)	10.213	7.66

*Though the vaccine received during the year 1987-88 is less than the number of beneficiaries, this is possible because of carried supplies of the previous year i.e. 1986-87.

Supply of measles vaccine by government and Rotary is as follows:

Year	Government	Rotary	Total
1987-88	540,000	384,000	924,000*
1988-89	1,184,500	1,118.450	
1989-90	1,193,500	400,000	1,593,500

The above explanation of the implementation is indeed a miracle when one considers that, in the fall of 1979, no organized program of immunization was in place in the state of Tamil Nadu. When one realizes the influence that the Rotary Club of Madras had on the health benefits for the children of the state it is purely miraculous. Let us never forget the power of dedicated Rotarians.

PDG Fred Black visited India as our volunteer on January 19, 1989. He returned home on February 4. He was disappointed not to witness the arrival of the 400,000 doses of measles vaccine, but Air India, once again, had still not committed itself to free air transportation. Fred reported that the measles program was alive and well despite the problems encountered during phase two. He also reported that the state of Kerala was finally coming around to the idea of agreeing to a "hold harmless" agreement.

The vaccine's free transport was finally granted by Air India on April 27, and arrived in Madras on May 29, 1989. Krish reported that there were some problems with clearance of the vaccine, and consequently it was lying in the Air India hangar for two days. He suggested that for the future the following practices be instituted: 1) The invoice and packing list to be sent to him at least a week in advance of shipment; and 2) A consignment note would accompany the vaccine, with one copy mailed to Krish. "This will enable us to prepare a letter of guarantee and a letter of authorization, so that the vaccine can be cleared as soon as it arrives," Krish concluded.

In June 1989, Eva and I were preparing for a trip to Geneva. On the agenda were talks with the International Red Cross Society and WHO, concerning our proposed blood transfusion project in Cote d'Ivoire, Burkina Faso, Sierra Leone, Ghana and Mali. Bill Irwin, another member of our club, and his wife, Marian, accompanied us; our reception was very cordial. Both the International Red Cross and WHO encouraged us to pursue our endeavors. Following our three days in Geneva, Eva and I flew to Vienna. There we rented a car and set off for Hungary, arriving in Budapest the day before the first Rotary club was to be rechartered behind the former iron curtain, by President Royce Abbey. The chartering itself was a closed ceremony, and very quiet and unpretentious. However, President Royce had invited us to join in the celebrations that were to follow, outside Budapest at Tuk.

Our next trip was to Abidjan, on September 13, 1989, to start our exploratory investigation and to secure commitments from the ministers of health, Red Cross officials and, most important, the local Rotary clubs in the respective countries. After receiving a positive response in Cote d'Ivoire, we went on to Accra, Ghana; Freetown, Sierra Leone; and Burkina Faso, ending up in Bamako, Mali. We arrived home on October 9, 1989.

On October 19, 1989, I received the following telegram from Krish: "Expecting measles vaccine clearance shortly. Reconfirm date of shipment in January acceptable. Our district conference on January 21st."

In our year-end report to Rotary International, we acknowledged that we still had 500,000 doses to ship to finish the project. We were anticipating a shipment of 300,000 doses in June 1990, and 200,000 more in the late fall of 1990, with an anticipated completion of the project in 1991.

Chapter 30

We were now approaching the final stages of phase two of our expanded immunization program of red measles.

I first suggested in 1985 that a phase two program should be implemented. There was considerable discussion on whether or not we should proceed with a phase two. I was affirmative that we should proceed, especially when the state government had agreed to become partners in sharing the costs. This was a very important and historic decision taken by the state government. I was able to convince the committee that we should proceed towards implementing a phase-two program.

Once it was decided that we would proceed, the committee, after receiving approval both from The Rotary Foundation and CIDA, established the time and date of the volunteers' visits. The committee suggested that I would be the last volunteer in order in order to collect all the essential information for our committee's final report. . The statistical and scientific epidemiological report, along with the history of the development of the infrastructure that started off with 68,000 doses in 1979 and finally immunized 5.5 million South Indian children fourteen years later, would be my responsibility.

I started to give a lot of thought as to how I would accomplish this most important task. One of my dilemmas was not only to collect all the scientific details and epidemiological data but to also properly prepare a list of the major Rotarians who had made this thirteen-year project viable.

Another concern I had was how to properly identify and thank those

· Epilogue ·

Rotarians, without leaving somebody out. Eva was a great help and I started to prepare the content of my final report well in advance of my anticipated visit to India in May 1993.

Our committee structure had become very loose. The chairman had designated the treasurer to act in his absence during the winter months while he was in Florida. I appreciated that the project was finally coming to an end. There was one more shipment of vaccine to be sent to Madras.

A letter from the treasurer indicated that he had ordered 300,000 doses of vaccine to be shipped to India at the end of February 1990. He also related that he would be the volunteer in September 1991.

The order had been confirmed with Krish Chitale. The treasurer suggested that the committee would not need to send a volunteer, as Eva and I would be in Madras at the time of the shipment.

In his letter, the treasurer emphasized that the committee was now approaching the end of the project. He further stated that funds were in short supply. He concluded that the CIDA holdback of funds would not be released until the following confirmations had been received by our committee:

1) that the State Government would participate by providing their share of the vaccine, in order to maintain the immunization program that was started in 1979;
2) that the reports had been filed on the various clinics that were held, detailing where the immunization took place. The reports were to cover not only the vaccine sent by our committee, but also the vaccine contributed by the state government.

There had been difficulties in the early implementation stages of phase two. It was now apparant that the last shipment of vaccine of January 1989 was starting to be used. Krish reported this to me in one of our biweekly telephone calls. We had kept in contact on a regular basis via telephone since December 1979. It was apparent that the immunization process would now pick up in earnest. This I assumed had been due to the political instabilities of the state government.

I had certainly recognized the government's difficulties earlier. However, these difficulties had been overcome with a great deal of work on the part of Krish Chitale and his committee. If this was indeed the case, then I could foresee that we would be able to ship the fourth and fifth installments of vaccine—300,000 doses—in September 1990.

The treasurer also mentioned to Krish that if the above planning came to fruition, he would be the last volunteer in September 1991, and this would conclude the project. Unfortunately, this had not been communicated to the rest of the committee, or to me personally, that he would be the last volunteer.

The Department of Civil Aviation approved the free transport of vaccine mid December 1989. The 300,000 doses were then ready to be shipped as previously planned for February 1991.

I was still under the impression that I had been delegated to be the last volunteer when the committee first met in phase two. I had planned to visit India to conclude my final report in either in the fall of 1992 or the spring of 1993.

Eva and I traveled to Madras in May 1991 to collect the valuable information required for our committee's final report. This report would include all of the epideminological data, govermental difficulties in this two-phased project, and their resolutions of these problems, and a list of the Indian Rotarians who had contributed for over 13 years towards accomplishing this "miracle." The documented statistics were collected and a prelimminary draft of my report was prepared.

However, phase two of the red measles immunization program came to an abrupt end. Unbeknownst to me and other committee members, the project terminated without any formal report from the committee. The remaining funds of the project, $6000, would be returned to CIDA and The Rotary Foundation. I was to learn about this decision in September 1993 when I received the final financial report. At that time I was preparing my final report which contained all the statistical, epidemiological evidence, changes in governmental attitudes, etc., in phase two. I had gathered all the information on my visit to Madras in May 1993. This information would have been extremely valuable in assessing our committee's fourteen-year involvement in the red measles immunization program in South India.

I realized that there would be no official and final document from our committee. All the necessary statistical data had not been collected. I felt that this approach was a tragic end to a project which I had been personally involved with since September 1979.

In conclusion, let me express again these thoughts which are always with me:

Ten children die each and every minute of every hour of every day, year in, year out, from communicable diseases that can be prevented by immunization. Five of these are from measles.

Another ten children become handicapped from communicable diseases that can be prevented by immunization, each and every minute of every day, year in, year out. Five of these are from measles.

Appendices

Measels Committee Structure 229

Volunteers 230

Receipts and Disbursements, Phase One 232

Receipts and Disbursements, Phase Two 234

Personal Disbursments, Phases One and Two 238

Bio-data, Kenneth C. Hobbs, O.Ont. MD 245

Measles Committee Structure

1979

Kenneth C. Hobbs, O.Ont MD, was asked by Rotary Governor Bud Crookes to initiate a 68,000 dose "red measles program" on behalf of Rotary District 7070 in conjunction with the Rotary Club of Madras to celebrate the International year of the child. He was accompanied to India by his wife Eva. This project was entirely financed by Rotary District 7070 with a matching grant from The Rotary Foundation, and a grant from The Canadian International Development Agency.

1980-1984

(Phase One—this phase was financed by a Health Hunger & Humanity grant from The Rotary Foundation, and the Canadian International Development Agency.)

Chairman	P.D.G. Paul McKelvey	Alliston, Ontario
Treasurer	P.D.G. Wilf Wilkinson	Trenton, Ontario
Secretary	P.D.G Fran Smith	Toronto, Ontario
Member	P.D.G Fred Black	Guelph, Ontario
Medical Advisor	Kenneth C. Hobbs MD.	Whitby, Ontario

1985-1993

(Phase Two—this phase was financed by a Health Hunger & Humanity grant from The Rotary Foundation, the Canadian International Development Agency, and by the State Government of Tamil Nadu South India,)

Chairman	P.D.G. Fran Smith	Toronto, Ontario
Treasurer	P.D.G Wilf Wilkinson	Trenton, Ontario
Secretary	P.D.G. Fred Black	Guelph, Ontario
Member	P.D.G. Paul McKelvey	Alliston, Ontario
Medical Advisor	Kenneth C Hobbs MD	Whitby, Ontario

Volunteers

1979 (September)　　　Kenneth C. Hobbs O.Ont MD,
　　　　　　　　　　　and his wife Eva *1

Phase One

1980 (October)　　　　Kenneth C Hobbs MD, and his wife Eva *1
1981 (January)　　　　P.D.G. Fran Smith (Toronto) and
　　　　　　　　　　　P.D.G Aubrey Oldham (Bracebridge)
1981 (September)　　　P.D.G Dave Theunessen (Swan Lake Man)
　　　　　　　　　　　and Alex Clough (Australia)
1982 (January)　　　　Kenneth C. Hobbs MD. *2 -
　　　　　　　　　　　P.D.G. Jack Laycock (New Brunswick) and
　　　　　　　　　　　Teddy Yamada (Japan).
1982 (September)　　　P.D.G. Wilf Wilkinson (Trenton Ontario)
1983 (January)　　　　P.D.G. Fred Black (Guelph On) and
　　　　　　　　　　　P.D.G. John Severs (U.S.A)
1983 (September)　　　Kenneth C. Hobbs MD, and his wife Eva *1
　　　　　　　　　　　P.D.G. Dave Kennedy (Guelph Ontario)
1984 (July)　　　　　　P.D.G Paul McKelvey (Alliston Ontario).
1985 (January)　　　　Kenneth C. Hobbs MD, and his wife Eva *3

Phase Two

1986 (January-February) Kenneth C. Hobbs MD, and his wife Eva *1
1987 (September)　　　P.D.G Fran Smith (Toronto Ontario)
1988 (January)　　　　Kenneth C. Hobbs MD and his wife Eva *4
1989 (January)　　　　P.D.G. Fred Black (Guelph Ontario).
1990 (January)　　　　Kenneth C. Hobbs MD and his wife Eva *1
1990 (September)　　　P.D.G Wilf Wilkinson (Trenton Ontario).
1991 (January)　　　　Kenneth C. Hobbs MD and his wife Eva *1

1991 (August)   P.D.G. Paul McKelvey (Alliston Ontario)
1993 (May)   Kenneth C. Hobbs MD and his wife Eva [1]

*1 There was no expenses either to the committee or Rotary International.
*2 The air flight was paid by The Rotary Foundation as Ken was a group study exchange team leader.
*3 The cost of his airfare was paid by the committee; however the cost of his flight was given back to The Rotary Foundation.
*4 The air flight was paid by Rotary International as he represented the president of Rotary International at two district conferences.

Rotary 3H Red Measles Immunization Fund—India
Phase One
Final Statement of Receipts and Disbursements
From Inception to March 15, 1985 (Canadian Funds)

Actual	Total	Budget
RECEIPTS		
Rotary International ($146,475 U.S Funds)	$181,507.00	$181,507.00
C.I.D.A	$434,430.00	$439,430.00
Interest earned and exchange difference - net	$88,528.00	$64,466.00
Other		$733.00
	$705,198.00	$685,403.00
DISBURSEMENTS		
Vaccine	$655,169.00	$634,375.00
Vaccine Guns	$4,759.00	$4,792.00
Volunteers		
Air transportation and travel costs	$24,372.00	$22,980.00
Unbudgeted items		
Contribution to report from India		$2,000.00
Purchase of film about project	$7,000.00	$9,000.00
	$704,137.00	$685,403.00

Excess of Receipts over Disbursements	$1,061.00
ADD: Amount receivable from C.I.D.A	5,000.00
surplus from project to be refunded	6,061.00

DETAILS OF ASSETS AS AT MARCH 15, 1985
CLOSE OF PROJECT

Bank Balance	$1,061.26
Amount receivable — C.I.D.A	$5,000.00
	$ 6,061.26

DISTRIBUTION OF REMAINING ASSETS

Rotary 3H	$181,507/ $615,937	$1,786.16
C.I.D.A	$434,430/$615,937	$ 4,275.10
		$6,061.26

NOTE: $5,000.00 would be deducted from C.I.D.A.'s distribution as these funds were not received. This would result in C.I.D.A. owing, as their final payment, $724.90, which would be paid to the Rotary International 3H Fund together with the current bank balance of $1,061.26 to provide them with their share of the surplus from the project which totals $1,786.16

3H Red Measles Immunization Program
Phase Two
Statement of Receipt and Disbursements
from Inception to February 4, 1994

DATE	EXPLANATION	RECEIVED $	DISBURSED $	TOTAL $
04/29/1986	FUNDS FROM R.I ($62,800 US)	$86,343.72		
05/23/1986	FUNDS FROM C.I.D.A	$61,700.00		
05/30/1986	BANK CHARGES			3.70
06/30/1986	BANK CHARGES			2.50
07/31/1986	BANK CHARGES			2.50
08/31/1986	BANK CHARGES			2.50
09/30/1986	BANK CHARGES			2.50
10/31/1986	BANK CHARGES			2.50
11/18/1986	INTEREST EARNED	3,296.84		
11/28/1986	BANK CHARGES			3.00
12/18/1986	CONNAUGHT LABORATORIES			62,500.00
12/31/1986	BANK CHARGES			3.00
01/15/1987	CONNAUGHT LABORATORIES - CH #3 ERROR IN DECEMBER 18, 1986 PAYMENT			2,700.00
01/30/1987	BANK CHARGES			3.60
02/27/1987	BANK CHARGES			3.00
03/31/1987	BANK CHARGES			3.00
04/30/1987	BANK CHARGES			3.00
05/11/1987	FRAN SMITH CH # 4 TELEPHONE, TELEGRAM & POSTAGE -323.03 TRAVEL ADVANCE INDIA - 500.00			823.03
05/12/1987	TEMPORARY BANL LOAN	1,000.00		
05/12/1987	RAMADA RENAISSANCE HOTEL CK #5 MEALS			84.92
05/25/1987	INTEREST EARNED- GIC- BANK OF MONTREAL	5,100.00		
05/25/1987	BANK INTEREST			11.54
05/29/1987	BANK CHARGES			3.60
06/09/1987	BANK MEMEO- REVERSE O/D CHARGE	6.00		
06/11/1987	REPAY TEMPORARY BANK LOAN			1,000.00
06/12/1987	BANK INTEREST			2.60
06/30/1987	BANK CHARGES			3.00
07/03/1987	FRAN SMITH CH # 6 REIMBURSE AIRLINE TICKET TO INDIA			3,525.00
07/31/1987	BANK CHARGES			3.00
08/31/1987	BANK CHARGES			3.00
09/23/1987	INTEREST EARNED	1,718.63		
09/30/1987	INTEREST EARNED	37.65		
09/30/1987	BANK CHARGES			3.00
10/08/1987	CONNAUGHT LABORATORIES- SHIPPING CHARGES			1,872.00
10/31/1987	INTEREST EARNED	383.55		
10/31/1987	BANK CHARGES			3.00
11/30/1987	INTEREST EARNED	350.23		

Date	Description	Amount	Amount
11/30/1987	BANK CHARGES		4.00
12/21/1987	INTEREST EARNED	2,340.00	
12/31/1987	INTEREST EARNED	374.72	
12/31/1987	BANK CHARGES		4.10
12/31/1987	REFUND- TRAVELL ADVANCE FRAN SMITH	279.44	
01/31/1988	BANK CHARGES		4.00
01/31/1988	INTEREST EARNED	370.53	
02/29/1988	BANK CHARGES		4.00
02/29/1988	INTEREST EARNED	343.25	
03/04/1988	FUNDS FROM C.I.D.A.	46,700.00	
03/31/1988	INTEREST EARNED	645.44	
03/31/1988	BANK CHARGES		4.00
04/15/1988	INTEREST EARNED	310.25	
04/30/1988	BANK CHARGES		4.00
05/31/1988	BANK CHARGES		4.00
06/10/1988	WHARTON RENAISSANCE MEETING		140.66
06/30/1988	BANK CHARGES		4.00
07/31/1988	BANK CHARGES		4.00
08/31/1988	BANK CHARGES		4.00
31/09/88	BANK CHARGES		4.00
10/17/1988	INTEREST EARNED	4,274.18	
10/31/1988	BANK CHARGES		4.00
11/30/1988	BANK CHARGES		4.00
12/19/1988	INTEREST EARNED	2,340.00	
12/30/1988	McKELVEY CH# 10 TRAVEL TO INDIA -F.BLACK		4,429.00
12/31/1988	BANK CHARGES		4.00
01/31/1989	BANK CHARGES		4.00
02/14/1989	INTEREST EARNED	3,888.45	
02/17/1989	INTEREST EARNED	236.71	
02/28/1989	BANK CHARGES		4.00
03/16/1989	INTERERST EARNED	1,000.34	
03/20/1989	INTEREST EARNED	131.01	
03/31/1989	BANK CHARGES		4.00
04/17/1989	INTEREST EARNED	1,110.01	
04/19/1989	INTEREST EARNED	142.94	
04/30/1989	BANK CHARGES		4.00
05/31/1989	BANK CHARGES		4.00
06/16/1989	INTEREST EARNED	2,125.37	
06/19/1989	INTEREST EARNED	296.63	
06/21/1989	CONNAUGHT LABORATORIES		72,400.00
06/30/1989	BANK CHARGES		4.00
07/26/1989	CONNAUGHT LABORATORIES- SHIPPING COSTS		2,020.55
07/31/1989	BANK CHARGES		4.00
08/31/1989	BANK CHARGES		9.65
09/29/1989	BANK CHARGES		4.00
10/31/1989	BANK CHARGES		4.00
11/28/1989	INTEREST EARNED	2,712.33	
11/30/1989	BANK CHARGES		4.00
12/29/1989	BANK CHARGES		4.00
01/29/1990	INTEREST EARNED	1,603.85	
01/31/1990	BANK CHARGES		4.25
02/28/1990	INTERST EARNED	684.51	
02/28/1990	BANK CHARGES		4.25

Date	Description	Amount	Amount
03/31/1990	BANK CHARGES		4.25
04/29/1990	INTEREST EARNED	1,413.71	
04/30/1990	BANK CHARGES		4.25
05/31/1990	BANK CHARGES		4.25
06/28/1990	INTEREST EARNED	1,505.61	
06/30/1990	BANK CHARGES		4.25
07/04/1990	CONNAUGHT LABORATORIES- VACCINE		63,000.00
07/04/1990	CONNAUGHT LABORATORIES - SHIPPING COSTS	1,509.06	
07/31/1990	BANK CHARGES	6.40	
08/27/1990	MCKELVEY TRAVEL- CH # 17 TRAVEL TO INDIA- W.J.WILKINSON	4,379.00	
08/27/1990	INTEREST EARNED	324.03	
08/31/1990	BANK CHARGES	4.30	
09/30/1990	BANK CHARGES	4.95	
10/26/1990	INTEREST EARNED	253.15	
10/31/1990	BANK CHARGES	4.25	
11/30/1990	BANK CHARGES	4.25	
12/31/1990	BANK CHARGES	4.25	
01/31/1991	BANK CHARGES	4.50	
02/25/1991	INTEREST EARNED	251.87	
02/28/1991	BANK CHARGES	4.50	
03/25/1991	FUNDS FROM C.I.D.A.	61,700.00	
03/27/1991	INTEREST EARNED	258.71	
03/31/1991	BANK CHARGES	5.25	
04/30/1991	BANK CHARGES	4.50	
05/24/1991	INTEREST EARNED	862.11	
05/27/1991	INTEREST EARNED	109.21	
05/31/1991	BANK CHARGES	4.50	
06/24/1991	INTEREST EARNED	385.22	
06/30/1991	BANK CHARGES	4.50	
07/26/1991	INTEREST EARNED	400.10	
06/26/1991	INTEREST EARNED	415.85	
07/31/1991	BANK CHARGES		4.50
08/19/1991	MCKELVEY TRAVEL TRAVEL TO INDIA- PAUL MCKELVEY		5,756.00
08/26/1991	INTEREST EARNED	402.65	
08/31/1991	BANK CHARGES		4.50
09/24/1991	INTEREST EARNED	194.77	
09/30/1991	INTEREST EARNED	356.79	
09/30/1991	BANK CHARGES		4.50
10/10/1991	CONNAUGHT LABORATOTIES- VACCINE		69,000.00
10/24/1991	INTEREST EARNED	92.27	
10/31/1991	BANK CHARGES		5.95
11/30/1991	BANK CHARGES		4.50
12/31/1991	BANK CHARGES		4.50
12/31/1991	BANK CHARGES		4.50
01/31/1992	BANK CHARGES		4.50
02/28/1992	BANK CHARGES		4.50
03/31/1992	BANK CHARGES		4.50

04/30/1992	BANK CHARGES		4.50	
05/31/1992	BANK CHARGES		4.50	
06/30/1992	BANK CHARGES		4.50	
07/31/1992	BANK CHARGES		4.50	
08/31/1992	BANK CHARGES		4.50	
09/30/1992	BANK CHARGES		4.50	
10/31/1992	BANK CHARGES		4.50	
11/30/1992	BANK CHARGES		4.50	
12/31/1992	BANK CHARGES		4.50	
01/31/1993	BANK CHARGES		4.50	
02/28/1993	BANK CHARGES		4.50	
03/31/1993	BANK CHARGES		4.50	
04/30/1993	BANK CHARGES		4.50	
05/31/1993	BANK CHARGES		4.50	
06/30/1993	BANK CHARGES		4.50	
07/31/1993	BANK CHARGES		4.50	
08/31/1993	BANK CHARGES		4.50	
09/30/1993	BANK CHARGES		4.50	
10/31/1993	BANK CHARGES		4.50	
11/30/1993	BANK CHARGES		4.50	
12/31/1993	BANK CHARGES		4.50	
		300,772.63	295,535.31	5,237.32

DETAILS OF ASSETS AS AT FEBRUARY 4, 1994

BANK BALANCE 5,237.32

Personal Disbursements—Phases One and Two

DATE	AIR FLIGHTS	HOTELS	MISC.	LOCATION	SUBTOTAL	TOTAL TO DATE
Sept-79 (to introduce measles vaccine to Madras South India. 100% volunteer)	$3,250.00 X 2	LONDON—3 NIGHTS @$250.00	FOOD $250.00	LONDON	$7,500.00	
		ROME—2 NIGHTS @ 350.00	FOOD $275.00	ROME	$975.00	
		BOMBAY 2 NIGHTS @ 150.00	FOOD $200.00	BOMBAY	$550.00	
		NEW DELHI 3 NIGHTS @$150.00	FOOD $195.00	NEW DELHI	$645.00	
		MADRAS HOME HOSPITALITY	FOOD NIL	MADRAS	NIL	
		HONG KONG 2 NIGHTS $150.00	FOOD $175.00	HONG KONG	$475.00	
		SIDE TRIP $11850.00 X 2		SIDE TRIP	$3,700.00	
					__$13,645.00__	__$13,845.00__
Mar-April 1980 (to work in Vietnamese boat camp Hong Kong 50% volunteer)	EVA'S AIR FLIGHT TORONTO TO HONG KONG $1,950.00	MARCH 1ST TO APRIL 20TH 1980 ACCOMMODATION'S PAID BY ROTARY FOUNDATION.	FOOD $1500.00	HONG KONG	$1,500.00 $1,950.00 __$3,450.00__	__$17,295.00__
Oct-80 (MEASLES India 100%volunteer)	$4500.00 X 2	FRANKFURT 2 NIGHTS @ 287.50	FOOD $235.00	FRANKFURT	$9,810.00	
		KARACHI 2 NIGHTS @ $200.00	FOOD $275.00	KARACHI	$675.00	
		NEW DELHI 5 NIGHTS @ 195.00	FOOD $520.00	NEW DELHI	$1,250.00	
		MADRAS HOME HOSPITALITY	FOOD NIL			
		BANGKOK 5 NIGHTS @ $300.00	FOOD $625.00	BANGKOK	$2,125.00	
		KHONG KONG 3 NIGHTS @ $245.00	FOOD $275.00	HONG KONG	$101.00	
		SAN FRANCSICO 3 NIGHTS @ $245.00	FOOD $550.00	SAN FRANCISCO	$1,285.00	
					__$16,155.00__	__$33,450.00__

Date	Details		Location	Amount	Total
Aug-81 (100% volunteer)	EVANSTON $850.00 X 2	Briefing for visit to West Africa as Pres. Stan McCaffrey's special representative			**$1,700.00**	**$35,150.00**
Sept-81 (3H polio project West Africa 100% volunteer)	$3850.00 X 2	ZURICH 2 NIGHTS @$225.00 DAKAR 3 Nights @ $275.00 BANJUL THE GAMBIA HOME HOSPITALITY FREETOWN S.L. HOME HOSPITALITY RABAT MOROCCO 3 NIGHTS @ 200.00 MEKNESS MOROCCO 2 NIGHTS @175.00	FOOD $235.00 FOOD $175.00 FOOD $75.00 FOOD $175.00 FOOD $125.00	ZURICH DAKAR BANJUL RABAT MEKNESS	$8,385.00 $1,000.00 $75.00 $775.00 $475.00 **$10,710.00**	**$45,860.00**
Oct-81 (100% volunteer)	EVANSTON $850.00 X 2	DEBRIEFING MEETING			**$1,700.00**	**$47,560.00**
Jan-Feb 1982 (GSE Team Leader to Dist 320 India and measles project)	AIR FLIGHTS PAID BY ROTARY FOUNDATION	LONDON 1 NIGHT PAID BY ROTARY NEW DELHI 2 NIGHTS @ $195.00 DIST 320 HOME HOSPITALITY BOMBAY 1 NIGHT @ $150.00 ZURICH 2 NIGHTS @$135.00	FOOD $75.00 FOOD $135.00 FOOD $75.00 FOOD $125.00	LONDON NEW DELHI BOMBAY ZURICH	$75.00 $330.00 $225.00 $395.00 **$1,025.00**	**$48,585.00**
Feb-April 1983 (boat project Medan Sumatra, Indonesia 100% volunteer)	$4500.00 X 2	TORONTO 1 NIGHT @ 135.00 LOS ANGELES 1 NIGHT @ 125.00 TOKYO 3 NIGHTS @ 375.00 HIROSHIMA 2 NIGHTS @$285.00 OSAKA 1 NIGHT @ $195.00 SINGAPORE 1 NIGHT @ $185.00 JAKARTA 5 NIGHTS @ 325.00 MEDAN 30 NIGHTS BISHOP'S HOME PARIS 1 NIGHT @ $175.00	FOOD $85.00 FOOD $105.00 FOOD $875.00 FOOD $325.00 FOOD $115.00 FOOD $145.00 FOOD $375.00 FOOD $125.00 FOOD $140.00	TORONTO LOS ANGELES TOKYO HIROSHIMA OSAKA SINGAPORE JAKARTA MEDAN PARIS	$9,220.00 $230.00 $2,000.00 $895.00 $310.00 $330.00 $2,000.00 $125.00 $315.00 **$15,425.00**	**$64,010.00**

Date / Notes	Ticket	Itinerary	Food / Notes	Location	Amount	Total
Aug-83 (measles—100% volunteer)	$4800.00 X 2	NEW DELHI 2 NIGHTS @ $195.00 MADRAS HOME HOSPITALITY AMSTERDAM 2 NIGHTS @ $155.00	FOOD $165.00 FOOD NIL FOOD $175.00	NEW DELHI MADRAS AMSTERDAM	$10,155.00 $485.00 $10,640.00	$74,650.00
Aug-84 (polio plus for Pres. Carlos Canseco MD)	EVA'S TICKET $4750.00 KEN'S TICKET PAID BY THE ROTARY FOUNDATION	ABIDJAN-COTE d'Ivoire - 3 NIGHTS ACCRA GHANA - 3 NIGHTS FREETOWN - SIERRA LEONE 3 NIGHTS BANJUL THE GAMBIA 2 NIGHTS	ALL ACCOUNTS PAID BY THE ROTARY FOUNDATION		$4,750.00	$79,400.00
Jan-85 (Ken's ticket paid by the Measles Committee The amount of the ticket was reimbursed to The Rotary Foundation—re: Paul Harris Fellowship for Susheila Chitale)	EVA'S TICKET $4800.00	NEW DELHI 2 NIGHTS @ $210.00 MADRAS HOME HOSPITALITY 3 WEEKS IN DIST 320 HOME HOSPITALITY BOMBAY 1 NIGHT @ 250.00	$4,800.00 FOOD $145.00 FOOD NIL FOOD $95.00	NEW DELHI BOMBAY	$565.00 $345.00 $5,710.00	$85,110.00
Jan-86 (family exchange & measles project 100% volunteer)	$3,300.00 x 2	LONDON 1 NIGHT @ $100.00 NEW DELHI 2 NIGHTS @ $155.00 AGRA 1 NIGHT @ $125.00 JAIPUR 1 NIGHT @ $110.00 MADRAS 4 NIGHTS HOME HOSPITALITY BANGALORE 1 NIGHT @ $125.00 MYSORE 1 NIGHT @ $125.00 OOTY 2 NIGHTS HOME HOSPITALITY COIMBATORE 2 NIGHTS FREE BOMBAY 1 NIGHT @ $145.00 ZURICH 1 NIGHT @ $115.00	FOOD $75.00 FOOD $135.00 FOOD $75.00 FOOD $85.00 FOODS NIL FOOD $50.00 FOOD $75.00 FOOD $85.00 FOOD $100.00	LONDON NEW DELHI AGRA JAIPUR BANGALORE MYSORE BOMBAY ZURICH	$6,775.00 $445 $200.00 $195.00 $175.00 $200.00 $230.00 $215.00 $8,435.00	$93,545.00

Date	Details	Locations/Nights	Food/Misc	City	Amount	Total
Aug-86 (3H project Singer Sewing Machine Co)	$2500.00 x 1 PAID BY ROTARY INTERNATIONAL	PEGASUS HOTEL 10 NIGHTS PAID BY THE ROTARY FOUNDATION		GEORGETOWN	NIL	$93,545.00
Sept-Oct - 87 (polio plus)	ALL COSTS PAID BY ROTARY FOUNDATION	ABIDJAN 3 NIGHTS—PDG CONSTANT ROUX GUINEA CONAKRY—3 NIGHTS ACCRA GHANA—3 NIGHTS LOME TOGO—2 NIGHTS YAOUNDE CAMEROON—3 NIGHTS DOULA CAMEROON—3 NIGHTS KINSHASA ZAIRE—4 NIGHTS NAIROBI KENYA—2 NIGHTS ANTANARIVO MADAGASCAR—4 NIGHTS NAIROBI KENYA—1 NIGHT KIGALI RWANDA—4 NIGHTS			NIL	$93,545.00
Jan-Feb 88 (presidential representative plus measles project)	PRES. KELLERS' REP TO DIST CONFERENCES 3100 and DISTRICT 3200 INDIA ALL COSTS PAID BY ROTARY INTERNATIONAL	NEW DELHI—2 NIGHTS MARADABAD—2 NIGHTS DIST. CONFERENCE MADRAS 8 DAYS MEASLES PROJECT COIMBATORE—3 DAYS MEASLES PROJECT OOTY—3 NIGHTS DISTRICT CONFERENCE BOMBAY—1 NIGHT			NIL	$93,545.00
Apr-88 (polio plus, site visit to Bogota Columbia 50% volunteer)	EVA'S TICKET—$2,800.00 KEN'S TICKET PAID BY THE ROTARY FOUNDATION	TRINDAD 1 NIGHT @ $175.00	FOOD $85.00	TRINIDAD	$3,060.00	
		GEOGETOWN GUYANA 2 NIGHTS @$155	FOOD $125.00	GEORGETOWN	$280.00	
		BOGOTA COLUMBIA—4 NIGHTS @ $220.00	FOOD $150.00	BOGOTA	$950.00 **$4290.00**	**$97,835.00**

Date	Cost	Itinerary	Food	City	Amount	Total
Aug-Sept 88 (blood bank project & 3H site visits 100% volunteer)	$5120.00 x 2	DUBLIN 2 NIGHTS @ $175.00	FOOD $210.00	DUBLIN	$10,800.00	
		IRISH TOUR FOR 7 DAYS BY CAR CAR $650.00 HOTELS $875.00	FOOD $675.00	IRELAND	$2,200.00	
		ABIDJAN-COTE DIVOIRE- 3 NIGHTS FREE	FOOD NIL	ABIDJAN		
		ACCRA GHANA 2 NIGHTS @ $150.00	FOOD $145.00	ACCRA	$445.00	
		FREETOWN SIERRA LEONE 2 NIGHTS $175.00 PER NIGHT	FOOD $135.00	FREETOWN	$485.00	
		OUAGADOUGOLU BURKINA FASO 3 NIGHTS @ $125.00 PER NIGHT	FOOD $210.00	OUAGADOUG.	$585.00	
		BAMAKO MALI 3 NIGHTS @ $185.00	FOOD $160.00	BAMAKO	$715.00	
		SEN MALI 2 NIGHTS FREE	FOOD $50.00	SEN	$50.00	
		DAKAR SENEGAL 5 DAYS @ $190.00	FOOD $350.00	DAKAR	$1,300.00	
		NOUAKCHOTT MAURITANIA 3 NIGHTS @ $165.00	FOOD $210.00	NOUAKCHOTT	$705.00	
		BANJUL THE GAMBIA 1 NIGHT @ $175.00	FOOD $100.00	BANJUL	$275.00	
		GUINEE BISAU 3 NIGHTS @ $125.00	FOOD $210.00	BISAU	$585.00	
		BANJUL THE GAMBIA 2 NIGHTS @ $175.00	FOOD $300.00	BANJUL	$650.00 $18,795.00	$116,630.00
Oct-88 (3H site visit 100% volunteer)	$2650.00 x 2	HOUSTON TEXAS 1 NIGHT @ 125.00	FOOD $55.00	HOUSTON	$5,355.00	
		MONTERREY MEXICO HOME HOSPITALITY	FOOD NIL	MONTERREY	$5,355.00	$121,985.00
Jun-89 (blood bank project visit to WHO Geneva & International Red Cross Budapest Charter of Budapest Rotary Club 100% volunteer)	$3,400.00 x 2	PARIS 1 NIGHT @ $185.00	FOOD $200.00	PARIS	$7,185.00	
		CAR TRIP THRU FRANCE, CAR $525.00 HOTELS $850.00,	FOOD $775.00	FRANCE	$2,150.00	
		GENEVA 2 NIGHTS @ $350.00	FOOD $375.00	GENEVA	$1,075.00	
		BUDAPEST 3 NIGHTS @ $285.00	FOOD $195.00	BUDAPEST	$1,050.00	
		CAR RENTAL $475.00		$475.00		
		VIENNA 1 NIGHT @ $165.00	FOOD $65.00	VIENNA	$230.00 $12,165.00	$134,150.00

Date	Amount	Details	Location	Cost	Total
Sep-89 (blood bank project research visit to Ministers of Health and Red Cross officials 100% volunteer)	$4,950.00 x 2	ABIDJAN COTE D'IVOIRE 3 NIGHTS WITH CONSTANT ROUX--HOME HOSPITALITY FOOD NIL ACCRA GHANA 2 NIGHTS @ $175.00 FOOD $145.00 FREETOWN SIERRA LEONE 3 NIGHTS $185.00 PER NIGHT FOOD $175.00 OUAGADOUGOUL BURKINA FASO 3 NIGHTS @ $130.00 FOOD $195.00 BAMAKO MALI 3 NIGHTS @ $185.00 FOOD $210.00 TOUR OF BRITTANY COAST $1500.00 FOOD $475.00 PARIS AIRPORT 1 NIGHT @ $175.00 FOOD $130.00	ABIDJAN ACCRA FREETOWN OUAGADOUG BAMAKO FRANCE PARIS	$9,900.00 $495.00 $730.00 $5,585.00 $765.00 $1,950.00 $275.00 **$14,725.00**	**$148,875.00**
Jan-90 (measles 100% volunteer)	$9,245.00 x 2	LONDON 3 NIGHTS @ $375.00 FOOD $275.00 MADRAS 20 DAYS WITH KRISH FOOD NIL LONDON 1 NIGHT @ $175.00 FOOD $85.00	LONDON MADRAS LONDON	$19,890.00 $260.00 **$20,150.00**	**$169,025.00**
Feb-91 (measles 100% volunteer)	$9245.00 x 2	TOUR BY CAR OF SOUTHERN ENGLAND FOR 10 DAYS TOTAL COST $2,650.00 MADRAS 21 DAYS WITH KRISH FOOD NIL LONDON AIRPORT OVERNIGHT @ $165 FOOD $75.00	ENGLAND MADRAS LONDON	$18,490.00 $2,650.00 $240.00 **$21,380.00**	**$190,405.00**
Jan-92 (site visit at no cost to the Newmarket Rotary Club Hospital Project 100% volunteer)	$2,345.00 x 2	TORONTO AIRPORT 1 NIGHT @ $165.00 FOOD $95.00 MOREILLA MEXICO 3 DAYS NO CHARGES		$4,930.00 **$4,930.00**	**$195,335.00**

April-May 1993 (final phase 2 of measles project-site visit and Melbourne Convention 100% volunteer)	$10,250.00 x 2	MADRAS FOR FINAL WORK UP OF PHASE TWO. 15 DAYS IN MADRAS, THEN ONTO CONVENTION IN MELBOURNE.	$20,500.00 $215,835.00
Oct-94 (earthquake site visit for the District Committee 100% volunteer)	$10,000.00 x 2	TO VISIT THE EARTHQUAKE SITE FOR THE DISTRICT COMMITTEE. RECEIVED TAX RECEIPT FROM THE COMMITTEE ACTUAL COST WAS $11,000.00	$11,000.00 $226,835.00

KENNETH C. HOBBS O.Ont. MD

EDUCATION:
   Primary and Secondary education in Ottawa Ontario, graduated from Glebe Collegiate June 1948.
   BA (Gen. Science) University Western Ontario 1951.
   MD Degree, University of Western Ontario 1955.
   Internship Ottawa Civic Hospital June 1955-June 1956.
   Residency in General Practice, Ohio Valley General hospital, Wheeling West Virginia 1956-1957.
   Cofounder of The Whitby Medical Center, July 1957.

COMMUNITY SERVICE:
   Member of the Whitby Public School Board 1959-1965, Chairman 1960-1965.
   Member Whitby District High School Board 1996-1997.
   Elected member of the Whitby Town Council, 1967-1975.
   Chairman of the site committee for The Whitby General Hospital 1959-1962, Chairman of the building committee for The Whitby general Hospital 1962-1970, Member of the board of Governors of the Whitby General Hospital 1966-1976, Chairman of the Board 1973-1976, Chief of Staff 1976-1979.

SERVICE CLUB SERVICE:
   Charter member of the Whitby Lions Club 1959-1961
   Member of the Whitby Kiwanias Club 1967-1970.
   Member of the Rotary Club of Whitby 1976 to present.

ROTARY SERVICE AT CLUB AND DISTRICT LEVEL:
   President of the Rotary Club of Whitby 1984-1985.
   Governor of District 7070 1985-1986.

ROTARY INTERNATIONAL SERVICE:

Introduced the first "red measles vaccine " into India September 1979.

Medical Advisor for the 3-H measles program "phase one"—1980-1984.

Medical Advisor for "phase two " red measles project 1986-1993.

Second World Wide volunteer for Rotary International to the Vietnamese Boat camps in Hong Kong March- April 1980.

Special representative for President of Rotary International Stan McCaffery to establish Polio projects in Morocco, Senegal, The Gambia, and Sierra Leone in September-October 1981.

First Medical volunteer to the Medan Sumatra Indonesian boat project March-April 1983.

Member of President Carlos Canseco'c committee to draft a program to eliminate polio by the year 2005. This project was called "POLIO PLUS".

Member of Rotary International "Health, Hunger and Humanity" committee 1985-1986.

Cross Canada Media Tour for The Rotary Foundation October 1986.

Co-chairman of Rotary International's Consultative Committee for Public Relations 1987-1988.

Consultant to the Programs Committee of The Rotary Foundation, 1987-1990.

Member of the founding committee for Rotary Volunteers in Action 1988.

Member of the Rotary Volunteers in Action committee 1991-1992.

Member of U.S.C.B Polio Plus Task Force 1993-1994.

Chairman of The Permanent Fund of The Rotary Foundation 1996-1999.

INTERNATIONAL PROJECTS DESIGNED BY KENNETH C. HOBBS O.Ont. MD.

- Red measles Immunization project in South India.1979-1993, 5.5 million children were immunized against measles. At a cost of $1.5 million US dollars.
- West Africa Brace Project 1983-1985, with a budget of $475,000.00. This project was designed to teach modern brace technology to Morocco, Senegal, The Gambia and Sierra Leone.
- Workshop for the Handicapped in Madras India, with a total budget $500,000.00.
- Supply of surgical equipment to the first non-profit pediatric hospital in south India. This was a 3-H project (Health Hunger Humanity) with a total budget of US $635,000.00.
- Literacy training project in Coonors south India with a budget of over $45,000.00. Over 2500 teachers have been trained to teach literacy, basic health, sanitation and cottage industries to women in the village areas.
- Water restoration project in Madras India, where 4 old Temple tanks were restored to act once again as reliable aquifers. The cost of this project was $50,000.00.
- A $500,000.00 US dollar project was approved in November 1997 to establish a Vocational and Rehabilitation Training Center in Madras India, where some of the 3 million disabled person who have had polio will be helped to walk and be trained so that they can become self reliant and sustained persons.

RECOGNITIONS:

- In 1984 a wing of the Whitby General Hospital was named after him in recognition of his service to the hospital.
- Citizen of the Year award was bestowed on Ken in 1990 by the Whitby Chamber of Commerce.

He was the recipient of the Commemorative Medal on the 125th anniversary of the Confederation of Canada, in recognition of significant contributions to Compatriots, Community and to Canada.

Meritorious Service Award from The Rotary Foundation in 1993.

Service Above Self Award from the Board of Directors of Rotary International, he was one of 94 to receive such distinction. This was awarded in 1994.

Third Level Gift award from The Rotary Foundation in recognition of Ken and his wife Eva's endowment fund of $250,000.00. This endowment has been dedicated to help improve the status of children in South India.

Ken was awarded the prestigious "Distinguished Service Award " from The Rotary Foundation in May 1997. No more than 50 Distinguished Service Awards are granted yearly.

On May 27, 1998, Ken was inducted with the "Order of Ontario" for his international humanitarian service.

The Rotary Foundation honored Ken as the first Canadian to receive, along with eight other Rotarians worldwide, the "POLIO PLUS PIONEER" award for his early work throughout the world in helping to irradiate polio. Rotary will have irradicated polio from the world by Rotary International's 100th birthday in the year 2005.

In December 1999, Ken was selected as one of the 100 persons who had made a difference in Durham Region in the past 100 years.

FAMILY:

Ken and Eva have been married for forty-six years. They have three children and four grandchildren.